The Healthcare Students' Academic Companion

The Healthcare Students' Academic Companion: An Aid to Effective Learning

Steven Moutrey

 Open University Press

Open University Press
McGraw-Hill Education
8th Floor, 338 Euston Road
London
England
NW1 3BH

email: enquiries@openup.co.uk
world wide web: www.openup.co.uk

and Two Penn Plaza, New York, NY 10121-2289, USA

First edition published 2020

A catalogue record of this book is available from the British Library

ISBN-13: 9780335249336
ISBN-10: 0335249337
eISBN: 9780335249343

Library of Congress Cataloging-in-Publication Data
CIP data applied for

Typeset by Transforma Pvt. Ltd., Chennai, India

Praise for this book

The Healthcare Students' Academic Companion: An aid to effective learning by Steve Moutrey.

I am Phil Ashwell (ODP) and many years ago was a student of Mr Moutrey. Ever since graduating we have always kept in contact or even worked together. We have the utmost respect for each other's attributes. Mr Mountrey has written this book for the students he teaches. He has written it with desire and passion, exactly the same way he teaches – always engaging. I have no problem endorsing this book as I will be adopting it into my own students reading list as I think it is simple to read, direct and very precise about academic skills. I believe there is a large market for this type of litera-ture as nothing has come out in recent years which is easy to follow and stay engaged with. I fully support and endorse this book.

Phil Ashwell MA (Ed) BSc (Hons) FHEA PgCert CODP HCPC
University of West London
Professional Lead for Operating Department Practice
Course Leader MSc Paramedic Science
College of Nursing, Midwifery and Healthcare

This book is certainly an ideal companion for any healthcare student as they initially commence and then progress through their course of study. Essential academic topics are explored within key themes and easy to read chapters. If you ever have the question 'what is meant by?' this book will certainly help in providing the answer and making sense of it.

Mike Donnellon
Senior Lecture in Operating Department Practice
University of Central Lancashire

Contents

List of Figures

Acknowledgements

Help and support from Dr Chris Markham, Head of School, School of Health and Care Professions, University of Portsmouth.

Mr Chris Wells, Allied Health Professions Lead, School of Health and Care Professions, University of Portsmouth.

Introduction

Education is a window – look through it to see where you're going

This textbook aims to aid healthcare students with clear and effective learning support, designed to help them understand the core principles, theories, skills and knowledge in education. It will enhance the learning experience so the student can apply it effectively and build on it, both in their initial studies and future practice. Supporting academic skills, allowing success in essay writing, research, reflection and critical appraisal, along with the need to understand evidence-based practice and its essential importance, this text provides the necessary knowledge and guidance to enable students to cope with the rigours of education required for successful completion of their studies prior to registration as a practitioner. Getting the best out of education will allow and ease the transition into the workplace with confidence, being fully prepared to meet the needs for continued learning and appraisal of relevant evidence and thinking to enhance practice.

Therefore, the book will also provide a supportive 'aide-memoire' to post-registration/qualified practitioners requiring a refresher in study skills if they are about to undertake further, post-registration studies to enhance and further their careers. It will also provide guidance for qualified, registered professionals, as all are required to continually learn and develop both skills and knowledge as their career progresses, and indeed as the requirement for re-validation comes around. There is information in this text that will help guide and inform all healthcare practitioners who are required to research, audit, write and learn for progression and career development.

A clinician is a professional who never gave up – life is a continuous learning cycle, gaining experience. You fail only if you give up and do not take advantage!

1 Making Sense of Essay and Academic Writing

Failure is not a problem, but failure to try will not be valued

So what's the problem?

In any course of Higher Education, students will always, and certainly at the beginning of their study, find essay writing an onerous and bewildering task. They will not quite grasp the rationale as to why it is relevant or required, seeing its production as a difficult task; as such, they will regard it as a 'must do', to pass the artefact of a particular module so they can progress as necessary. The majority of students feel this way, so you will not be alone in this train of thought. However, you can do it! No one will tell you it's going to be easy; gaining your chosen award was never going to be easy, and as an undergraduate student the thought of your journey towards your degree has, no doubt, had some trepidatious moments when you consider, 'was this the right thing to do?' Hopefully, though, you will have a certain passion for the field and topic of study, especially as it will lead to a specific, planned end point: a career and employability, which will bring their own rewards. These rewards will, positively, motivate you to the final achievement and the end of the course.

One of the things to keep in the back of your mind about essays is the fact that in your chosen field of practice or career, you may be required – or indeed 'want to' – write reports or articles for publication. It may come as a surprise that undertaking essay writing at any stage of your chosen degree or study will be good practice for when you 'have' to produce these reports or write articles for publication based on ideas and research identified to enhance your knowledge and understanding as a practitioner in a career and employment.

So, as essay writing is a common, if not mandatory, feature of any undergraduate study in all facets of healthcare specialisms, you will need to relate to the epistemological scaffolding of work, information and validity of evidence that constitutes effective knowledge and quantifiable information. Epistemology, which will be covered later in the book, is the process of knowing 'how and what' we should know, based on how and what we 'actually' know – so, to briefly summarize: the theory of knowledge and what justifies 'us' knowing and believing, individually, what we do.

One method to overcome your immediate 'blank' or trepidatious thoughts about how you should begin the essay writing process, is to get a blank piece of paper and write down any 'things' that bother you about beginning an essay or assignment – as in the box below:

Things that bother me are:

You may be surprised by some of the thoughts that come to the fore – things such as:

- What is meant by the learning outcome I have to write about?
- I don't know what to choose as a topic!
- Am I going to cover the topic well enough?
- I don't know where to start!
- Are my spelling and grammar good enough?
- How am I going to contain all the information in the given word count?
- Am I going to write enough to meet the word count?
- Where am I going to find enough references?
- Have I got enough time?
- What tense do I have to write it in?
- How do I reference it?

These provide just a few examples of the 'oh, my goodness, how do I start' thoughts you may have. But it's a good start, as it begins to focus your mind on the way

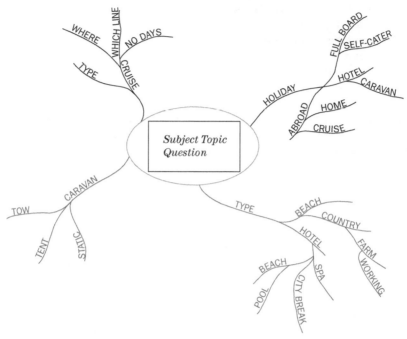

Figure 1.1 Example of a mind map

forward – and from small acorns grow large oaks! This forms the start of one tech-nique that can be used to begin your essay planning – the thought shower. Starting with your given topic or specific learning outcome at the centre, start pulling out ideas and concepts that are linked and that you may want to include, or use to describe/expand on the original topic or question. 'Teasing' these out from your central 'hub' will start to develop other ideas and ways ahead. The 'mind map' is another similar tool that can be adopted (Figure 1.1). This, like the thought shower, is a simple but powerful tool that can help in mapping your thoughts into a logical sequence, enhancing your problem solving and helping you formulate a plan to follow, and giving structure to your first thoughts on planning the essay.

Now delve deeper into the main title, highlighting subtitles or topics, then add further, smaller lines that extend from each subtitle. Continue this until you have definitive tasks or ideas that will inform the way in which you should focus on infor-mation you need to acquire. This will give you the direction of your essay and what you need to achieve to address the subject area or topic. The following suggestions will give you early ideas of how to progress your 'mind map' and inform the varied 'branches':

1. 'Free write' about the subject
2. Analyse the question
3. Mind-map the topic areas

4.   Identify areas to read about
5.   Select literature
6.   Read the selected literature critically
7.   Make notes and continue researching
8.   Plan citations to use
9.   Start writing

Always bear in mind that an academic essay is a written source of communication. It must be clear, concise, well organized and coherent, and above all must be understandable to the reader.

Theory

Theory is important to grasp in the writing of any essay, as the theoretical alignment of any healthcare practitioner or student will inform the various routes of questioning required to look at the ways in which their evidence is sought and gathered. What needs to be grasped is that any essay in healthcare is governed by the importance of using sound research that informs evidence-based practice – evidence that goes to support and inform sound clinical practice. An understanding of the arguments based on 'theory' is paramount to the provision of knowledge, which will lead the writer to justify and engage in healthcare-related areas being scrutinized.

Critical thought and argument need to be evaluated, and the various theories behind any piece of research that will inform your own essay will need to go through this process. Theories can be used to inform, support or conversely invalidate any question or research outcome, and therefore require careful consideration before inclusion in your own work. The value judgements you make about what you read need to inform and validate your own question, and this will need to be reflected in your writing – critical appraisal of all relevant information will need to be reflected in your work, highlighting theory, both good and that which may be unsubstantiated. What is important in essay writing in the health sciences is that sound, well-researched evidence is paramount in supporting arguments and theories – both of which may have some impact, ultimately, on patient outcomes and care.

Choosing the topic or addressing the given learning outcome

This is the point where you need to make a decision – either on addressing a given learning outcome or choosing a topic for research or a specific article you'll need to write about.

This is the first stage where you ask the following question: How does my essay plan, thought about to this point, relate to the essay question or topic title? This will not be the only time you need to ask this question – it's one that you constantly need to revisit at every stage of your essay production to ensure you remain on the right track.

This is all about the planning of your essay and I would suggest that the following guide will give you a systematic approach to this:

1. Carefully look at the learning outcome(s) or topic – don't move on until you fully appreciate what it means and what you need to do.
2. Make relevant notes about the topic and 'mind-map' the title.
3. Ensure you understand how this fits into the module you're undertaking or the area of research you are about to undertake.
4. Consider your knowledge: is it adequate to address the subject appropriately? If you need to do more reading around the subject, do it now before moving on.
5. Understand the language of the question/learning outcome – unpick the various meanings: 'concept' words give you the meaning or topic issue you need to write about; 'procedure' words will give you the tasks, i.e. 'explore', 'discuss' or 'evaluate'. These will give you the direction in which you will need to answer the particular 'question'.

If you're about to undertake a research topic, then you will need to start thinking about the methodology – this is covered in Chapter 3, 'Research Methodology: What Is It and What Is the Potential?' This applies to everything, whether it's an essay you are writing or a research article for publication. It also applies equally to writing a report – although depending on the subject of the report, your approach may need to fit the report title – but the same thought principle will still apply.

Stages of production

The writing process, broadly, has three main stages. By following these stages you will have a structure that will hopefully inform all the essential requirements of the work. They will ensure that you are working logically, to a set method that gives you the required accuracy in production.

Figure 1.2 will show a brief methodology to follow.

Preparation

You will by now have thought about the topic or specific learning outcome you are required to focus on. By using the above stages, you can now start to think about the process of writing and beginning the essay. At this stage, you will now start to look at key words – having read around the subject and formulated a 'mind map' of where you need to focus, key words will have been identified. These will help to identify the topic or issue you need to write about, and some common words will become familiar:

- **Analyse**   Look at the issues; examine the various parts and examine each issue, highlighting its relevant relationship.

- **Argue**   This is where you state your case based on the evidence researched and the work sequencing around your discussion.
- **Compare**   Talk about the similarities between different characteristics and qualities highlighted from your reading into the subject.
- **Contrast**   Evaluate and discuss the differences between the characteristics.
- **Critique**   Make a judgement after analysis of your findings, giving examples, looking at the positives and negatives based on the criteria.
- **Describe**   Talk about and write about the various features and qualities of the topic.
- **Evaluate**   Look at and discuss the various arguments, reaching a significant judgement around the values of your research.
- **Interpret** Discuss what you mean in relation to the specific topic and outcome.
- **Justify**   Provide a rationale for a particular course of action, attitude or methodology.
- **Prove**   Demonstrate your logical approach and argument.
- **Summarize** In brief, give a precise description of your findings and conclusions.

The preparation stage will give you clarification around the discussion, explaining and even rethinking the assignment question to enable full understanding of the outcome required. You will by now have an understanding of the proposed structure and question to be answered. The content and length of the essay should have been

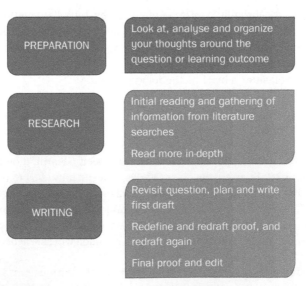

Figure 1.2 Stages of writing

addressed and you'll have an idea of exactly how much time is required to complete both research/reading and the writing itself. At this stage, if more clarification is required, then now is the time to seek advice – this can be gained in consultation within your peer group, if appropriate, or by seeking specifics from the tutor/lecturer or co-writing colleagues. It's now time to move on and start dedicated reading and research into what you need to fully inform your writing.

Critical thinking

Making sense of the topic and/or the question to be addressed should now be foremost in your mind. Behind this, though, is the need and ability to think critically about what you need to address in your writing. The aim of this is to provide an objective and evaluative source of thought to enable a judgement to be made. You must be able to link any and all connections between any concepts you have discovered up to now in both your planning and reading. Do your thoughts convey a logical message that you wish to highlight in your planning, and will this progress into a 'flow' and sequential, logical progression in your essay? It is essential in any social or healthcare science to be able to 'think critically', logically and make sense of other eminent writers, authors and facilitators who have contributed in the area being addressed. Certainly, the need for close interrogation of their work and publications is paramount: this can only add value to your own work. Making sense of an argument or discussion, evaluating whether something is correct or an accepted practice, is a good thought to always have in the back of your mind. This leads you down the path of questioning, finding a connection between what you have read and what you think, looking at the variations and differing component parts of the available data.

This can be quite a complex activity as trying to make sense of an argument will hopefully allow a concise and logical approach to finding answers to questions you may have in respect of your own hypothesis or question. The 'Mapping knowledge, theories and concepts' model (Figure 1.3) may help you to focus on this area of your discussion and put it into context, guiding you through the process.

When searching for relevant information to use in your assignment (or writing/production of any kind) to endorse your own argument – i.e. a reference – having some form of algorithm may help. You will need to critically analyse the reading of any article to make that informed decision as to its appropriateness to your own discussion. Does it appropriately define a position you need to address? Does it define relevant terms and information that back up your own ideas and thoughts? This is where critical thinking is important, along with understanding of where the article fits into your own patterns of thinking. You will by now have read around the subject comprehensively and narrowed down the relevant from the not so relevant. You should now be confident that you have useful sources of text that can be dovetailed into your own work to reinforce your argument and discussion. The main point of this process is to obtain information that will enhance critical thinking, help with your analytical processes, summarize your thoughts around information that

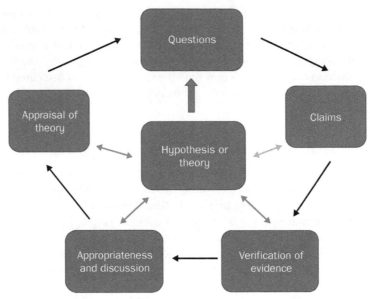

Figure 1.3 Mapping knowledge, theories and concepts model

is essential and focus on any and all philosophical principles that underpin the thoughts and arguments to be used in your assignment or production.

Critical thinking may well be described as an 'ableness' to reason, engage and connect various ideas in a logical fashion through reflection on a given subject – the ability to question rather than accept anything at 'face value'. The skills required for anyone to arrive at the best possible outcome and solution to an issue can be described thus:

- Observe and understand links between ideas
- Establish the importance and evaluate differing ideas
- Understand and appraise various opinions
- Identify contradictions and irregularities in reasoning
- Systematically evaluate problems in systematic process
- Inform and justify reflection on the given situation and your own assumptions

Within critical thinking there are times and events that may influence the way we (critically) think which is not diagnostic, analytical or impartial. It is human nature to have certain emotions that may affect our objective decision-making – anger, joy, grief or anxiety – which may be due to many influences on our psychological state of mind at the time. An awareness of this as a potential problem and one which may affect our critical reasoning is important to consider.

As you, as a healthcare practitioner, progress through your career, critical thinking may well prove to be a key attribute that your employer or organization requires; it may well form part of the job description for a role that you aspire to move into. Promotion and direction of career 'travel' may require you to own such skills to enable you to fulfil that role, and you may need to emphasize these skills, either through the application or interview process. The interview process may include some form of hypothetical scenario which you would be required to talk through, and this will probably involve some form of critical thinking. You may be expected, or even wish, to become involved in research, audit or even writing reports – all of which will require some form of critical thinking.

Another cogent example of critical thinking may require you, for example as the ODP team leader in a specific operating theatre and its proposed list, to use critical thinking skills to analyse the caseload, operating list running order and organization to enable the best treatment order, to formulate that list making best use of all resources available to maximize the best utilization and patient throughput.

So, in summary, this is a skill that is aimed at:

- achieving the best outcome of a given situation by obtaining all relevant information and evaluating the outcome by looking at all possible sources of information
- developing your foresight to make best decisions without 'outside' influences affecting that decision, by gathering all relevant information and synthesizing the strengths, weaknesses and all possible impacts it may have on the outcome

You must also ensure that a review is undertaken to analyse the impact of change, if this is the outcome. Probably the best way to achieve this is by reflection. You may want to reflect on the whole process and its outcome to see if further change needs to be implemented. Reflection will be covered in depth in Chapter 2.

Research

Research methodology, or search strategy, which will be fully covered in Chapter 3, now needs to be identified. However, at this stage you will need to read within a broad field of previous papers, in journals and texts. This will start the information gathering process. Always keep the specific assignment question in the back of your mind so as not to 'wander' off the subject area.

By this stage you will have formed a good understanding of where you need to go, having now gained an understanding of the topic. Focus on detailed reading around the subject, which will give you an idea of how to address your line of writing, answer and perspective around your argument.

Validation is now the key word – you will have a good line of enquiry which will identify your subject outline and allow you to apply the detailed reading to inform and qualify statements in your essay – so you are writing from an informed perspective. You should now be in a good position to have a clear idea of where you need to go! You should have formulated a clear view and set a logical plan around your argument and focus.

Writing

Now is the time to consider your plan of writing. After organizing yourself and the reading you have undertaken, identification of the research methodology or search strategy, if applicable, and the particular format you wish to use, the first draft is now ready to be written. This is the time to plan, draft, redraft and revisit the question. The redraft will probably be the main focus of your writing and will no doubt throw up more questions and the need for further reading and research around your given question. This will further strengthen your argument and provision of evidence, allowing a more coherent approach prior to the final draft and edit, making the structure into a sound and flowing essay.

Proof and read for grammar, punctuation and spelling, getting an independent person to also read and proof your work – someone who is not necessarily an expert in the subject but can give constructive feedback about the layout and how the essay flows. By now you will have put the essay or assignment into its required layout and logical sequence. You will, no doubt, have taken the opportunity to submit a draft to your tutor for comment! Take careful note of feedback and amend as appropriate. If this possibility does not exist and you are writing as a qualified practitioner, utilize the expertise of a fellow colleague or practitioner. All constructive feedback is incredibly important.

Structure and layout

This very much depends on the type of essay or assignment you are writing – it could be a report, feedback on a project, an audit or an article based on a research-related topic, and you will need to identify this in the layout.

Does it need an abstract? Or does it just need an introduction which highlights the topic being discussed? The following will give an overview of a typical layout which will cover most academic writing, be it an essay, assignment or academic paper.

Title – Include your name, course name and course title and the essay question or learning outcome(s) in full.

Abstract – If required, this will need to present a concise overview of the content of the work and what was achieved, the methodology and a summary of the outcomes. Normally this would be the last thing written after the main body and assignment have been completed.

Introduction – Set the scene! The introduction will provide an interpretation of the essay/assignment title, the parameters and issues forming the main focus of the particular examination of the topic or question. It will contextualize these parameters, as well as particular practices, research and any theoretical issues and principles. If it has any link or relevance to your particular practice, this should be highlighted here.

Main body – This will show the evidence, including the presentation of empirical data and a critical overview of the relevant literature, duly referenced. All relevant issues in the differing contexts, debates and even controversies would be included within the main body. This is where, if appropriate, you would include up-to-date material from your own perspective or experience if it links in with the topic being discussed. This must be clearly differentiated from the material derived from other sources.

Within the main body, your analysis of evidence derived from research and bibliographic reading would be set out. The following approaches could be looked at for inclusion, depending on the type of presentation being written:

- Consideration of coherence and clarity of reading for completeness
- Addressing critical questions as they arise (or not)
- Compare and contrast with relevant evaluations, which would look at similarities between different characteristics
- If relevant, the inclusion of results from evaluative frameworks, and the application of theoretical models and principles
- If appropriate, this is where you would report on the use of analytical tests carried out

Your writing should focus on presenting paragraphs that are clear and balanced. A good rule to adopt is keeping each paragraph to a set number of sentences, which are succinct and to the point – this will reduce the risk of 'waffling' and so distracting from the salient points required to address the topic. Keep the number of sentences to three or four only, as this will provide a sense of cohesion. With every focused point raised with your paragraphs, you should be drawing closer to finalizing the indicative impetus behind the essay. Your academic essay is a tool used to transfer ideas, beliefs or statements about your particular topic or learning outcome. This should lead the reader towards a similar level of comprehension regarding the subject to yours, and as you near the end of the main body, this should be moving towards your conclusion.

Ensure that all relevant information is appropriately referenced in your text (see 'Referencing' below). Use of pronouns such as 'I', 'you', 'we', 'they', 'our' or 'your' should be kept to a minimum in most academic subjects. Some institutions will only accept essays written in the 'third person'.

Conclusion

To make it a success, by this point, your essay should have provided all relevant information to meet the need – whether it's a question or learning outcome, have these been answered? The conclusion should now provide a reminder to the reader of what the essay is about and what has been achieved. The conclusion must therefore provide a summary of what has been stated, its relevance to the subject area

PREPARATION Research and plan the essay
TITLE State the learning outcome, question or topic
INTRODUCTION Description of the situation or topic Explanation as to what is to be achieved and the specific situation
MAIN BODY Presentation of the main information and research to meet the question or topic Support with articles, examples or evidenced ideas Evaluation of research and/or ideas
CONCLUSION Clear relationship to learning outcomes or question with summary of data Implications or outcomes Further reading or research recommendations

Figure 1.4   The structure of an essay

and whether there is any specific connection to a personal or social/clinical context. What is important is to leave the reader with a strong statement that is going to impact on their comprehension.

The conclusion should enable the reader to clearly relate to the outcomes and analysis derived from the essay title and question. It should discuss the implications of any specific statements made and, if pertinent, give recommendations for further reading or research to progress the question or topic.

In summary, then, the basic structure of an essay is as shown in Figure 1.4.

Essay errors – common mistakes

Having now looked at various artefacts of the essay, perhaps now is a good time to look at some errors that are easy to make in its production. So what can commonly go wrong that reduces impact, flow and validity?

Some of the common areas that students and practitioners make mistakes in, are failing to adequately answer a question or learning outcome; misreading or failure to understand the desired outcome and going completely off the academic 'road' to meet this outcome. Some questions will demand a wide debate and discussion around a particular question or route of study with which you will need to

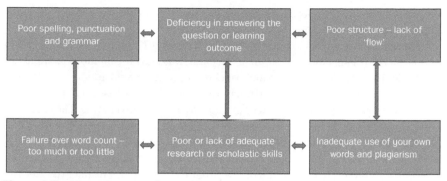

Figure 1.5 Common errors in essays

review and produce sound reasoning, but as the work progresses and the writing continues, the student may start to stray away from the chosen route of information required. This will then fail to connect to the debate being sought; constant reading and review of the work being produced will help to avoid this, along with utilizing the most relevant sources of information and understanding of the vast range of sources available. Other common errors can be summarized as in Figure 1.5.

Referencing

Referencing is used to give intellectual credit to the author of the source. It helps the reader recover sources quickly and easily and shows the amount of rigour undertaken to qualify reasoning and information in an essay or assignment. It also helps to avoid being accused of plagiarism. It is a method used to demonstrate that you have conducted a thorough and appropriate search of the literature, acknowledging that ideas and material that you have used in your own work belong to other authors. It is crucial to reference correctly and appropriately as it ensures that you have carried out relevant research around your specific topic or question, research project or academic paper. There are many styles of referencing, but with all of them there are two parts – citing and the production of a reference list. This is important as you should include all the sources that you use when creating a piece of your own work.

If traditional academic essays or assignments are to be sound and objective, it is important to use as up-to-date information and research as possible. First, it is of vital importance to identify the source or origin of the information used to qualify an argument. You may wish to use quotes in the essay. If quotes are cited, then quotation marks must be used and the author's name, the year of publication and the page number for the text of the quote must be included. Even if this information or quote is paraphrased – i.e. the author's original text has been rewritten in your own words – then the author's name (surname), the year and page number must still be included. If a brief summary is used in your text, or a general idea taken from an author, then an in-text reference needs to be provided giving the author's surname and the year only.

Generally there are two main types of reference used in universities: Harvard APA (American Psychological Association) and Vancouver. Common examples of use are in the sciences, education and psychology which would advocate the use of Harvard APA. This style is probably the most commonly used, especially for university students. Schools of law would normally use the Vancouver style. These are not prescriptive though, and may vary between different institutions.

Vancouver referencing is based on a numerical referencing style commonly used in medicine, and consists of citations which are numbered sequentially, linked to a reference list at the end of the paper or document. The list provides full details of the relevant and corresponding texts mentioned in the paper or document. So each particular piece of work cited should have a unique number attached to it, used in sequence throughout the whole piece of work. The number can be written in brackets at the end of the citation or it may be written as superscript. If a piece of work is cited more than once, then the same number should be assigned to the citation each time. If several pieces of work are cited in the same sentence, you will need to include the citation number for each reference; the following is an example where works 7, 8, 9, 18 and 20 have been cited in the same place in the text:

> *Several studies (7 – 9, 18, 20) have examined the effects of laminar flow within an operating theatre in a suite of operating rooms.*

Harvard referencing is used when directly quoting or paraphrasing a source, and would be located in the text of the essay as a fragment of the full citation/reference.

In-text citations may look similar to the following:

> '*I removed a part of the colon after it was found to be necrotic, which required an end-to-end anastomosis. . .*' (Morrow 2014).

The reference list is located at the end of the paper and will display the full citation from the relevant source used within the paper. An example of this would be:

> Morrow, R. (2014). *Surgery for Necrotic Bowel Syndrome*. New York: Whitley.

In general, Harvard reference lists of citations will follow the following format:

Name of author
Year published
Title
Place of publication
Publisher
Pages used

The citations in the reference list are formatted in alphabetical order by author's surname.

Do you need to consider ethical issues when writing your essay?

Whether or not you consider the issue of 'ethics' in your essay very much depends on what you write about, what type of work you are producing and whether it is based on research. Normally an academic essay written as part of a degree course, or similar, will not need ethical consideration. However, if you're attempting to write a research paper or dissertation, this may well be something that needs to be considered in the context of the research you are undertaking. Often, the individual who is attempting a research topic will spend time focusing on their work and what they want to achieve from the research, but they never consider its effect on the specific areas of research and its impact on other people. It is important to always bear in mind how data is collected and whether it is ethically sound, and that it should cause minimum harm to anyone who takes part or provides this data.

The simple explanation as to what, in this situation, ethics means in an educational context, is concerned with 'right' and 'wrong'. These issues of right and wrong, and how they are applied to educational research, become important as they need to be taken into consideration within the work or topic you are writing about. Ethics are important in this context as they provide a framework around moral principles and conduct, and what these have to do with the topic being addressed. This becomes an issue when you consider the work undertaken by others that you are quoting and using in your work to back up your argument. You cannot use the work of others unfairly, as if you do, it may be construed as injurious to them, and also their work being quoted or paraphrased may be misconstrued or taken out of context.

The basis of ethical principles to bear in mind can be described as suggested by:

- Proposal: what are your intentions?
- Potential: what are the benefits of your research?
- Permission: who do you need to gain access to or approval from?
- Protection: how will you ensure research participants and/or the organization are protected? How will you ensure that you are protected?

These principles will form the basis of your ethical considerations to avoid making procedural ethical mistakes.

Many aspects of writing and research require consent from the participants involved and who are active within the process. Their cooperation is required, whether they are individuals or specific institutions or organizations providing facilities, time or active involvement. Those involved may be exposed to risk, either emotional or physical. Obtaining their agreement is called giving 'informed consent'. This is an issue of 'freedom' within the rights of the individuals concerned as we live in a 'democracy' where their freedom of expression and 'speech' is an accepted norm and any infringement must be justified and consented to. Also, this has to be justified because consent before, during or after the 'event' or use, may be withdrawn. This becomes a consideration, as it will be seen as informed refusal to take part at any stage of the writing or research involvement.

So any research undertaken must be assumed under a common accord with all parties concerned, and therefore consent should be obtained within a contractual basis. Full information should be proffered to the various parties involved, giving a breakdown of the aims, objectives, how the research is to be undertaken and the nature of expected outcomes and procedural processes. What you don't want is to place barriers in the way and perhaps prejudice any results by withholding relevant information from anyone involved.

This is a brief description of the 'ethical' considerations when undertaking academic or socio-scientific writing or research. The following are considerations in summary of the type of information that should be considered:

- Anonymity needs to be offered and given to all participants
- Information gathered must be treated with confidentiality
- Consideration of the findings and final reports should be given to participants
- Give any interviewees the opportunity to see any findings or written statements before submission
- Seek permission from participants through a written, formal approach/ contract
- Inform all parties involved what will be done with the information provided
- Consider providing a written 'thank you' to all involved in the project
- Articulate why you are doing this research – is it for a degree course or other purpose? – state your hypothesis if necessary
- Consider the need to submit a proposal to an ethics committee for formal approval

Is the essay now complete?

The bulk of the hard work should now be complete and your 'scaffolding' has now been built on! This is a good time to review the work and add/remove the small nuances that will make a good essay into a great essay!

Reflect on the writing process just undertaken and ask yourself the following questions to refresh your mind on what you started out to achieve:

- Has the fundamental question or topic been addressed?
- Has this question been answered appropriately and to my satisfaction?
- Has the relevant material researched been comprehensive and up to date?
- Did the essay plan work and address the need?
- Are the researched references and bibliography annotated correctly and in alphabetical order?

- Have I shown use of academic skills in handling any relevant theory-to-practice links?
- Have I discussed the essay content in my own words and expressed ideas and arguments in my own words?

Once all these questions have been asked and addressed, now is the time to check some of the basic fundamentals:

- Have the grammar, spelling and punctuation been checked and proofed?
- Have I received relevant tutor feedback after submitting a draft?
- Is my word count/limit correct – within the regulatory boundaries?
- Most assignments or essays need to be double spaced with a font of 12 points – is there a minimum/mandatory margin requirement?
- Is there a requirement for a separate title page, and if so, what's required?
- Is everything included in the title page that is laid down by the institution?
- Can it be submitted electronically – if so, am I aware of the processes?

So, if everything has been thought through and all the questions have been answered, you can stop writing! You should now have full confidence in your work and be able to think back to the start of the process and say: 'I now don't have a problem!'

Further reading

Lee, K.C., Goh, H., Chan, J. and Yang, Y. (2007) *Effective College Writing: A Process Genre Approach*. Singapore: McGraw-Hill.

Redman, P. and Maples, W. (2017) *Good Essay Writing: A Social Sciences Guide* (5th edn). London: Sage Publications.

Soles, D. (2005) *The Academic Essay: How to Plan, Draft, Revise and Write Essays* (2nd edn). Bishops Lydeard, Somerset: Studymates Publishing.

2   Reflection and Reflective Practice

Reflection is the cornerstone of professional practice, providing the strength from which to build knowledge and innovative proficiency

The healthcare practitioner profession is demanding and involves complex interactions with patients and staff on a daily basis while in practice. These considerations may – and will – be forgotten in the daily rigours of practice, and cannot always be seen at first glance, as a result of the nature of our work. This is true both as a student and as a qualified registered practitioner.

For example, with regard to the profession of Operating Department Practice (ODP), strong, cogent skills are required not only from students but also from qualified, registered practitioners to enable the continuation of the care and support required to our patients who need surgery. Constant evaluation and development of skills and knowledge are paramount in our ethos of practice; the registering body – the Health and Care Professions Council (HCPC) – clearly states in the Standards of Proficiency (SOPs) for ODPs: *'Be able to reflect on and review practice'* (HCPC 2014, SOP 11, p10). The SOPs extrapolate this in sections 11.1: *'understand the value of reflection on practice and the need to record the outcome of such reflection'* and 11.2: *'recognise the value of case conferences and other methods of review'* (HCPC 2014).

Reflection is a well-used and useful tool to enable both understanding and evaluation of what, as healthcare professionals, we need to achieve and continue to learn, to improve the care we afford to the patients we deal with on a daily basis. Another specific concept in learning and development, it's another way (and a useful way) for professionals to learn from their experiences to develop and enhance team and personal practice. Irrespective of where we start to reflect, or what experience or subject we are reflecting on, the role of the practitioner and his/her thoughts on the subject will always be very personal, with personal and unique interpretations of the subject or experience. What is required is a suitable model that we, as professionals, can use to reflect by gaining best knowledge and understanding of a typical situation, and this can then be used to learn from and enhance progress and innovation. Adopting a notion of self-knowledge throughout a reflection and using an experiential learning cycle will provide an objective, strength-based approach which will put the experience into context; simply asking the following will provide the basis of a reflective account:

- What is reflection?
- Why do I need to reflect?
- Is reflection important in healthcare?
- Is it important for patient care?
- How can this improve my practice?

These points can be used first in a cyclical model (Figure 2.1), which will 'set the scene' and prepare a practitioner to undertake reflection by using a recognized model of reflective practice. Using this as a tool, leading back to the question of 'what is reflection?', will aid logical planning and thought into revisiting the notion of why it becomes important for each practitioner to plan appropriate care, using reflection to learn from experience and act on resultant actions.

Using this cyclical model and answering the specific questions can be helpful if a diary of practice is kept: a journal, in which notes are made of specific, interesting or, conversely, distressing experiences. This may help to focus on the ultimate reflection and its benefit both personally and in a group or team situation. Importantly, it may highlight that the reflective process doesn't necessarily need to be an individual or a singularly personal process. Group or team discussions become a source of experiential and intellectual support and learning for a given situation – important within the operating theatre team, when a debriefing after an event can become both psychologically and motivationally important to aid the 'moving on'

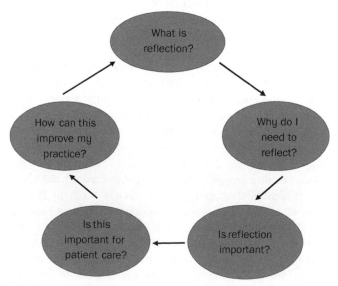

Figure 2.1 Reflective preparation cycle

from that experience, enhancing understanding. The spoken reflection, discussed amongst the various professionals involved, can be extremely important to support improved practice and emotional understanding.

The notion of reflection is generally understood to be based on a learning experience. It is useful to think about it as a learning cycle such as the experiential learning cycle provided by Kolb (1984). Kolb provided a framework of experiential learning, using a cyclical model in which one could organize a personal account, where the differing steps taken could be placed within a learning model or reflective experiential framework. So to answer the 'what' question, the practitioner needs to identify and understand (probably by personal analysis) the situation that has arisen as a result of experiential practice and observation – be it a good experience or a poorer one. Kolb's revised edition (2015) keeps the main text of his first book intact, which preserves the original statement of *Experiential Learning* in the theoretical state that was first alluded to.

The follow-on from 'what' therefore is 'why'. Why do I need to reflect? This part of the cycle has to come from some form of analysis of a given experiential situation. You will need to determine exactly what that situation has generated and how it fits within your healthcare practice. Your analysis will change over time as you gain experience and knowledge – a greater understanding and focus will become more apparent for you as an aspiring practitioner, offering different levels of appreciative perspective for any given event. This will lead you into a field of thought that will narrow your thoughts into a more competent and rational understanding of the particular issue that requires reflection. You will move on from a generalist approach, to specifics that fit the reflective needs and will give a more coherent approach to the issues of importance. This will help you, as a practitioner, to become more acutely aware of any beliefs, assumptions, conventions and norms that may have coloured your thinking in the early days of practice. We therefore reflect to enhance and progress practice and patient care in response to particular occurrences, to ensure better treatment, care and practice, acting to improve our future practice towards those we care for – our patients!

Is reflection important in healthcare? This is the next question that importantly impacts on the practice of the ODP (or any other healthcare professional).

Reflection is viewed as a strategy that is and remains important as an aspect of 'lifelong learning'. As we work in an ever-changing sphere of professional practice, that has the additional caveat of development and innovative growth in medical knowledge and which is required to continually enhance healthcare practice, we as practitioners need to embrace this development. The ever-increasing demand and requirement for all healthcare professionals to prove, through either revalidation or re-registration, that their 'continual professional development' (CPD) meets scrutiny and analysis of current practice are inherently important and are one area where reflection is vital. Reflection is one tool that can be employed to meet this requirement. It can be used to show how practice and knowledge meet the requirements, that as a practitioner you have remained up to date and have current knowledge of developments that have been made in healthcare practice to benefit patients and their care. This shows how it is important for patient care.

Does it improve my practice? This is a question that can be asked in many ways, highlighting the benefits of reflection: What are the benefits? What activities do I do that will promote and increase my knowledge? A number of areas can be highlighted with questions and debate to further the understanding of relevant issues:

- What motivates me as a practitioner?
- Do I understand the concepts and perceptions relating to best patient care?
- What are my feelings around specific issues?
- How can I compartmentalize these issues – do I need to?
- Do I adopt the correct attitude with regard to the required values?
- Can I differentiate between habitualization and the need to progress?
- Are my observations and conclusions going to both benefit the team dynamic and be accepted?

These are the questions that every professional in healthcare should be asking to plan actions and continually monitor and evaluate the quality of care that should be provided to every patient.

As with most theories and practices, there are going to be opposite and contrary ideas and limitations. These limitations may include:

- Lack of understanding – unsure of the process
- How do I undertake a reflection – what experiences are important to reflect on?
- Have I got the time required to undertake this?
- Knowing why reflection is undertaken – what is the benefit?
- Is a reflection going to be important to me and others – are they going to take note?

Concerns will surface if a reflection is done badly and the whole point is missed, as it shows an ineffective approach to the experience. The reflection may raise issues around practice that may not be seen as good, and possibly even reinforce bad practice by not being critical enough. This will lead practice to remain the same, and allow a cultural collusion to continue. If the reflection allows this, it will provide assumptions that all is well and no change is required. If this situation is allowed to thrive in practice, then it will exacerbate an inappropriate use of reflective practice, which will only serve to devalue the practitioner's work instead of promoting and changing practice positively (Quinn 1988/2000).

Activities to promote reflection are now being incorporated into undergraduate, postgraduate and continuing medical education across a variety of health professions (Mann et al. 2007). These activities are important as artefacts within (students') practice outcome documents as a tool to evaluate the achievement of learning and understanding in the practical fields of study.

Models of reflection

The need to look at the 'ways and means' of reflection at this stage is vital. It is important to follow a suitable method to aid your reflective practice and make sense of the
situation in a coherent and logical way. This will allow understanding, presentation
and further development and progression in learning to further your practice. It will
also allow you to bridge the theory–practice gap and understand the uncovered
knowledge in and on action (Schön 1983). Schön is probably the most prominent
name in reflective practice; he emphasized the need for reflection both 'on' and 'in'
action. On-action relates to the reflection on an experience that takes place after it's
happened, looking at the event you've been involved in and what you can take away
from it, positives and what could have been done differently. In-action is reflection
taking place at the time of the experience, reflecting on actions as they occur.

Borton's model

This model of reflection describes three basic premises:

What? – This will describe what happened, what happened to you and/or others:
What did I see? What did I or others involved in the particular event or issue do?
How did I or others react to this situation?

So What? – This is where you will evaluate and analyse the situation or event, ask
yourself why it happened this way and try to make sense of the issue. How did
this event make you feel? Once this has taken place, you need to ask yourself
about specific feelings – how do you feel now after the event in comparison to the
way you felt at the time of the event?

Now What? – This section needs to take into consideration any actions that are
deemed necessary based on what has been described in your analysis. What are
you, or others, going to do now as a result of your analysis, and how will these
issues be tackled and actioned?

Figure 2.2 shows one of the very early models of reflection as devised by Terry
Borton, from his book *Reach, Touch and Teach* (1970). Borton was an American
schoolteacher who showed a simple learning cycle asking three questions: What?
So What? and Now What?

Many students (or qualified practitioners), who find themselves needing to
reflect for the first time, find this an easy model to follow. Originally used in education, it's been latterly used by other practitioners outside this field. Healthcare practitioners, ODPs and nurses, in particular, find this an easy model to follow and use
for their reflections, as it lends itself to a process of practice based firmly on and
within experiences. The 'what' can be used to analyse a situation or event, with the
'so what' answering the question(s) raised as a result – allowing a knowledge base
to be formed. The 'now what' can then be related to how this new knowledge can be
used for improvement and advancement (of care) (Rolfe 2014).

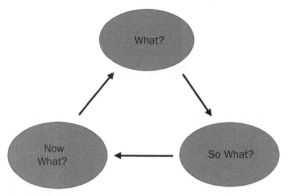

Figure 2.2 Borton's model
Source: Borton (1970)

An example case study of a reflective account using Borton's model under-taken by a first year operating department practitioner (ODP) student shows how this model can be used to good effect at the beginning of practice and study. It shows an early day's reflective account of an event that proves how useful reflective practice can be even during this early stage.

Reflections on professional practice

Introduction

Reflective practice can be used as a tool in practice-based learning. Reflection as described by Jasper (2003 p.99) is a method through which we can learn from our experiences. My reflection is based on an event that occurred during the third week of my second placement in the first year of my BSc (Hons) Operating Department Practitioner (ODP) degree course. Using Borton's frame-work model of reflection (Joyce 2014, p.119), I will use the three guiding questions from the model to structure my reflection, to focus my learning and provide a greater insight and understanding of the experience.

What?

The aim of the second placement was to build on my knowledge gained during the previous placement period and to enable me to learn new skills in the perioperative environment.

During the third week of my placement I was working with my mentor in the recovery room in order to gain a better understanding of the day-to-day, rou-tine patient care tasks undertaken. As part of the recovery team I was assist-ing my mentor to receive patients into the recovery area from the operating theatre team. On this particular occasion I was in the recovery bay awaiting the next patient whilst my mentor was completing some paperwork at the desk. Our patient arrived with the surgical team who began the handover without waiting for my mentor to arrive. As a student I asked them to stop and wait for my mentor to arrive, stating that I was not qualified to take the handover unsupervised at this stage of my training. The anaesthetist said that they thought that as I had confidently taken handovers previously when my mentor was present, I was more than capable to do so unsupervised. I explained to them that I knew the limits of my practice and as such was not able to take the handover without my mentor's presence, as set out in the Health & Care Professions Council (HCPC) Standards of Proficiency – Operating Department Practitioner (HCPC 2014, p.7, SoP 1.1). I went on further to explain that the reason for this was that during the handover, which they had started, were references to the patient's pre-existing medical conditions including diabetes and hypertension, that required additional tests which meant that we need to be extra vigilant within the handover provided to ensure that we carried out our duty of care in the best interests of the patient as per HCPC 2014, p.7, SoP 2.1 and 2.9.

When my mentor returned, the surgical team completed the handover to both of us and left us to recover the patient. Once the patient was responsive, we needed to carry out a number of tests including a blood sugar test and red blood cell count. Before carrying these tests out, my mentor introduced me again to the patient and asked if she had any objections to me assisting in the taking of blood samples for the tests. As we were going to be touching the patient, it was important to gain informed consent from them which I need to do at all times as set out in HCPC 2014, p.7, SoP 2.7. Having obtained the blood sample and results, we needed to check the dressing on the patient. As a female patient having undergone a gynaecological procedure, it was going to be an intimate examination and, as such, the lady may have felt uncomfortable with a man being present. In order to maintain her dignity, I explained to her that while my female colleagues carried out the examination I would step out of the bay and close the curtain.

So What?

After the series of events I reflected and discussed them with my mentor. She said that I had acted correctly when I had asked the anaesthetist to wait for her to arrive before taking the handover as I had demonstrated that I knew the limits of practice, as set out in the Standards of Proficiency HCPC 2014, p.7, SoP 1.1. As a student one can often be called upon to carry out tasks which are not within your scope of practice; by having the courage to speak up, I was able to also maintain a high standard of personal and professional conduct (HCPC 2014, p.7, SoP 3.1).

When working with service users it is also important to recognize that relationships should be based on mutual respect and trust (HCPC 2014, p.7, SoP 2.4). The events of this day highlighted the importance of respect for the service user. By taking into consideration the gender of the patient, I was able to provide a solution that helped them maintain their dignity and at the same time act professionally as set out in section 3.1 of the HCPC 2014, p.7, SoP.

During my placement within the recovery team the importance of maintaining own health as set out in the HCPC 2014, p.7, SoP 3.2 was also highlighted. Whilst on placement a member of the team developed a stomach bug which resulted in the individual feeling unwell during the course of the day. Due to the severity of the illness the member of staff left, as staying could have passed on the illness to service users as well as other team members. As an ODP it is important to remember that failure to maintain one's health and thereby fitness to practise can have serious consequences not only for the practitioner but also for service users you come in contact with.

Now What?

By reflecting on the events I have recognised and understood the importance of the Standards of Proficiency and how they impact colleagues and service users. From the events of the day I need to continue to speak up when I am asked to carry out tasks that are outside my scope of practice but at the same time ensuring I maintain a professional duty of care and always acting in the best interests of service users.

Conclusion

Having used the reflective framework by Borton I was able to analyse my reflection effectively in a structured manner and to identify how I could improve patient care in the future. The experience and subsequent reflection have helped me recognise and understand the importance of the Standards of Proficiency within the perioperative environment.

References

Health and Care Professions Council (HCPC) (2014) *Standards of Proficiency for Operating Department Practitioners*. London: HCPC.
Jasper, M. (2003) *Beginning Reflective Practice: Foundations in Nursing and Healthcare*. Cheltenham: Nelson Thornes.
Joyce, P. (2014) Reflection for Operating Department Practitioners, in H. Abbott and H. Booth (eds) *Foundations for Operating Department Practitioners* (pp. 109–124). Maidenhead: Open University Press, McGraw-Hill.

Reproduced by kind permission of Mr Noel Kithake, first year ODP student, University of Portsmouth (2017)

Gibbs' model

Another commonly used model in the field of healthcare practice is Gibbs' reflective cycle (Figure 2.3). This reflective cycle has become one of the accepted models

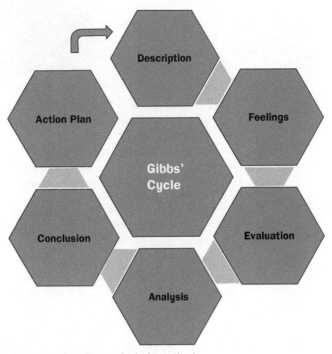

Figure 2.3   Gibbs' reflective cycle (adaptation)

to use in nursing and other professions allied to healthcare. Adapted originally from Kolb's experiential learning model – learning through experience – Gibbs' model is referred to as an iterative model, which means learning through repetition. Gibbs, an American psychologist and sociologist, published his reflective model in his 1988 book, *Learning by Doing*, which extols the systematic thinking around the experience a person encountered or endured during a specific event or activity.

Gibbs' model recognized six stages in the cycle:

- **Description** (of what happened)
- **Feelings** (what were you thinking and feeling at the time?)
- **Evaluation** (what was good and bad about the experience?)
- **Analysis** (what sense can you make of the situation?)
- **Conclusion** (what else could you have done?)
- **Action plan** (if it arose again, what would you do?)

This reflection process follows the six steps in order, so that each step or phase of reflection follows on and informs the next stage. There can sometimes be confusion over the analytical stage, as this is the only one that is not seen as a practical or experiential stage, as it requires a notion of thought analysis required to put into perspective the outcome of the incident or experience. The reflector may become confused and think of the evaluation, analysis and conclusion parts of the cycle as asking similar questions, which results in some form of analysis taking place, leading to repetition of information and thoughts. The analysis of the experience should only happen in the 'Analysis' stage – the other five stages are only to be used as 'statements' showing description, summative appraisal and statements of the justification of why something was done (or not), practically.

This model has proved useful in healthcare as it will (if used correctly) enhance personal self and self-improvement; it will link theory to practice, challenge your perspectives, and help to explore new ideas and innovations to improve a situation and how you as a practitioner will think about practice in the future. The fact that this is an acceptable model to use in practice can be seen by some as making it inappropriate for other situations, as it does not lend itself as a model where reflexive and critical approaches are required due to its simplistic format – it may not allow movement beyond practice principles. Explore values and have practice 'lead to change, commitment to quality and respect for difference' (Finlay 2008).

Johns' model

Designed by Christopher Johns, this model provides a structure to reflection that allows for a deeper and greater knowledge of the practitioner to be considered. The reflection process is designed to enable the practitioner to focus on an experience or situation and what has been learned, through sharing with colleagues or mentors. This process allows an experience to be looked 'into', gauging your own thoughts, emotions and feelings against looking 'outside' at the specific experience and situation, taking into account any wider perspectives and the consequences of any actions taken. These are the fundamental considerations that are suggested by Johns within the first two stages.

There are five stages described by Johns:

- Description
- Reflection
- Influences
- Evaluation
- Learning

The influences are about what, as a practitioner, 'influenced' your actions. Did you apply your expertise and knowledge, alongside previous experiences to the actions taken in this situation? Were there any ethical considerations to be taken into account? What other (if any) external influences did you need to consider?

In the evaluation stage, you would need to consider whether this situation was handled correctly and whether it could have been handled better. Consider whether there was significant impact on you or your patients, colleagues or other service users. Now would be the time to look at what 'learning' is required and, by reflecting on the situation, what you as a practitioner need to consider. What have you learned from the situation? Do you need to identify specific learning needs as a result of the experience, and is this something that the team needs to consider corporately?

So how do we reflect?

In the past (and sometimes still) reflection has been associated with education and not really considered in many other aspects of life. As healthcare providers, we should fully understand the benefit of this style of learning. Simply looking at and repeating what you have done and seen in practice (clinical or otherwise) and other situations will not be beneficial to you as a healthcare professional – it will not increase your effectiveness, as each situation you experience would not constitute a learning and developmental evolutionary experience. These situations and experiences may be unique but will not increase the effectiveness of your practice unless you 'do' something with them. You will only gain from the experience by undertaking some form of reflection and becoming a reflective practitioner.

As a student, it is becoming standard practice to produce reflections which can be assessed by means of individual pieces of work or separate artefacts within your learning progression. As a qualified practitioner, your effectiveness in practice will be assessed both by you as an individual and by others, especially in a team situation, with appropriate development resulting from good reflective practice. As a registered practitioner, reflection represents a record of what you have learned and how you have learned from a myriad of sources that will inform your practice in how you will do things differently in the future. The Health and Care Professions Council (HCPC) expects a registrant to 'be able to reflect on and review practice' (HCPC 2014, SOP 11). It also states that you need to 'understand the value of reflection on practice and the need to record the outcome of such reflection' (HCPC 2014, SOP 11.1). This ensures that the registering body for our profession checks on the practitioner's fitness to practise and maintains professional competence. There are a number of ways in which we can do this:

- **Reflective log (diary) of events and experiences**
  A reflective diary or log of events can include all aspects of what happened, what went well, what did not go so well and how this will influence future practice, to show what has been learned from that particular situation – this is where your chosen model of reflection will inform writing and future performance. It will allow the development of your analytical skills and inform judgements which will help to formulate well-informed decisions. There are a number of ways in which this can be achieved as a diary of practice: keep a record of the work undertaken; note existing skills you presently own, those you develop as a result and new skills learned; and identify areas you wish to improve.

- **Reflective portfolio**
  Similar to the diary, a reflective portfolio will show evidence of what you have learned from an event and how you have learned by it. Through the

content, it should demonstrate the evidence, with all necessary comments you feel appropriate to inform your future practice and how you came by this evidence.

- **Serious or critical incident**
  Any incident that could be classed as critical should have a reflection undertaken to highlight and identify the specifics of the incident. You would highlight the learning point of this and why it has been important to you as a practitioner. The main focus of this is what you have learned as a result of reflecting on the event. Don't fall into the trap of thinking that only negative experiences require a critical reflection – positive experience are just as important, especially when showing the learning points.

The benefit of being a reflective practitioner is therefore that it aids you in putting the experience into perspective, enabling learning to take place. This is very much a part of 'cycling' around the typical 'Kolb's Learning Cycle' (Figure 2.4), allowing us to think through a situation appropriately.

It may be useful at this stage to look at some terms and definitions that may help with the correlation of thought towards the process of reflection and how we may mind-map it in the early stages, helping to put the experience into a reflective, logical thought process.

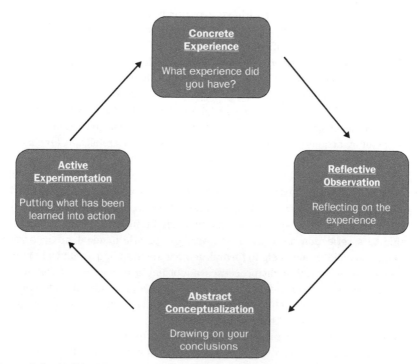

Figure 2.4 Kolb's adapted Learning Cycle

Identification of pattern: In cognition the identification or recognition of pattern may be something that is worth considering. It identifies a process where we can match information against particular stimuli or events that have informed us in the past; it can be matched from information that is already incumbent in our own memory or from experiences of others that have had an impact on us personally. Recognizable *patterns* may come from the understanding of a set of characteristics or features that either describe a situation fully or a process that has had a multitude of theories, processes or approaches without a definitive conclusion. Identification of a pattern may not happen immediately but it is usually linked to a gestalt or spontaneous thought that will have impact.

Interaction: A reaction between people or 'things'. Communicative interaction may be the foundation of why a reflection needs to take place – the foundation of why the experience requires to be reflected on. Examples may be:

> The theatre team leaders are not interacting enough with the clinical staff working on the theatre floor.
> There is good interaction between clinicians and the theatre staff by including all within the Multi-Disciplinary Team (MDT) meeting.
> The mannerism of the surgeon doesn't allow good interaction between himself and the patient, not allowing them to understand each other.

Interaction may feature strongly in any reflection as it may be the causative action necessitating reflection, or it may have a major influence on the reflection as a whole. It may have an impact on the conclusion, action or learning process required as a result of the action identified.

This fits well when considering **management and leadership**: being able to strike a balance between interpersonal skills is vital when dealing with various people within a team. This means having the knowledge of how they interact in a given situation, and balancing this against the specific fluency of 'expert' skills held by various people in various hierarchical posts. This is important to consider, as it may have dynamic consequences in future actions or recommendations resulting from a reflection. Preconceived individual ideas will proffer behavioural and predetermined ideologies because of learned life experiences. These may be difficult to overcome, but can be addressed by critical reflection on a situation by involving leaders and managers, and indeed senior clinicians in the decision-making process – team working and collaboration.

Insight: An intuitive understanding of a situation or experience may give direction to a reflection on a given scenario or specific incident or occurrence. Insight into an incident may help to formulate an understanding around a particular experience and inform thought processes accordingly to a relevant relationship that has influence on the incident or experience. It may provide an understanding of the motivational forces behind any actions that have occurred, the thought processes or the behaviours that have taken place.

Capture: There will be many artefacts that will need to be taken into consideration for any reflective account or interpretation of a given situation. It becomes important as to how we 'capture' these to put them into a logical sequence to enable full understanding, and how it will become a learning event. We need to capture the 'experience' – how we think, how we evaluate the various points for consideration. This also involves evaluation and consideration of 'right and wrong' – categorizing events and contextualizing them. The events and intricacies of the occurrence requiring reflection all need to be captured and placed into a logical sequence to allow full understanding and progression throughout the 'cycle' of reflection.

Summary

This chapter has hopefully provided you – the student, registered practitioner or indeed the educator – with a toolkit to progress the reflective skills required to build on your toolkit as a healthcare professional in practice. Reflective practice is therefore relevant to both the student in education and to the qualified practitioner, in practice. By using experiences and observations in the perioperative settings in which we work and practise, we can develop and further the knowledge that allows best practice and ultimately better patient care.

Simply, you 'do' something, think about the action and then decide on the best action and reaction to progress knowledge and understanding – importantly, not forgetting to include and evaluate your own feelings and emotions and how these have influenced you. In this way you can then map out clear progress as you learn and develop new skills to improve any given clinical experience as a healthcare practitioner.

References and further reading

Borton, T. (1970) *Reach, Touch, and Teach: Student Concerns and Process Education*. New York: McGraw-Hill.

Finlay, L. (2008) Reflecting on 'reflective practice'. PBPL. Paper 52, pp.1–27. Retrieved from: tinyurl.com/finlay-PBPL (Accessed 9 June 2017).

Gibbs, G. (1988) *Learning by Doing: A Guide to Teaching and Learning Methods*. Oxford: Oxford Brookes University.

Health and Care Professions Council (HCPC) (2014) *Standards of Proficiency for Operating Department Practitioners*. London: HCPC.

Jasper, M. (2003) *Beginning Reflective Practice: Foundations in Nursing and Healthcare*. Cheltenham: Nelson Thornes.

Kolb, D.A. (1984) *Experiential Learning: Experience as a Source of Learning and Development*. New Jersey: Prentice Hall.

Kolb, D.A. (2015) *Experiential Learning: Experience as the Source of Learning and Development* (2nd edn). Upper Saddle River, NJ: Pearson Education Ltd.

Mann, K., Gordon, J. and MacLeod, A. (2007) Reflection and reflective practice in health professions education: a systematic review. *Advances in Health Sciences Education*, 14(4): 595–621.

Quinn, F.M. (1988/2000) Reflection and reflective practice, in C. Davies, L. Finlay and A. Bullman (eds) *Changing Practice in Health and Social Care*. London: Sage [original work published in 1988 and reproduced in 2000].

Rolfe, G. (2014) Reach touch and teach – Terry Borton. *Nurse Education Today*, 34(4): 488–9.

Schön, D.A. (1983) *The Reflective Practitioner: How Professionals Think in Action*. New York: Basic Books.

Sherrat, N., Goldblatt, D., Mackintosh, M. and Woodward, K. (2000) *An Introduction to the Social Sciences: Understanding Social Change, Workbook 1*. Milton Keynes: The Open University.

3 Research Methodology: What Is It and What Is the Potential?

Knowledge is not measured by what we know, but how we seek and utilize it

Roots of research

Research and the term 'research' may, to some, be a tricky and fearful concept to grasp. It could be seen as having to learn a whole new language, with new concepts that are obscure and accompanied by whole new sets of jargon and vocabulary which need to be grasped before full understanding is achieved. This shouldn't be the case and certainly should not be believed based on a fallacy and mistaken assumption that it's beyond the ability of most practitioners in healthcare. Quality has got to be one of the most important issues to be addressed when thinking about research; research is about gaining new and meaningful knowledge and taking that knowledge, allowing it to impact on everything we do in practice.

Is research something that you feel is important for you solely to undertake to pass your degree or satisfy the need for a particular course outcome? If you think beyond these requirements and consider the true potential of doing research, you may feel that any research undertaken could help towards a contribution to the improvement of a particular situation, or betterment of a process – a process that may require development to make it easier or more understandable to implement, to meet the needs of new thinking or better the process. This should be the motivator for you when you consider and think about 'research'. A simpler way of thinking about research is that we all undertake it (probably without thinking) in everyday life. When shopping, for example, we look for the best products at the best price, looking at what's available both in the shops and online to get the product that best fits our needs and our 'pocket'. We undertake research when preparing for an interview; we look at the company or organization we are looking to join, to ascertain information we may need so that we can answer interview questions. Obviously there are many variants and differing concepts, constructs and methods to consider, but it will always offer the reward and outcome we look for and hypothesize over; ultimately, it will give us the new knowledge we require to further our understanding in whatever walk of life we follow.

Research is a systematic investigation into study in order to establish facts and reach conclusions. It will look at situations where we can make improvements, or offer new thinking around taking a situation forward into a new process to make a difference. Is healthcare at the pinnacle of its development and innovation, with nothing else that can be done to improve it? And is education the best it's ever going to be, to deliver the best knowledge possible in the most constructive and understandable manner?

If the answers to these questions are 'no', then you have the answer to why research is important and why it's undertaken – something you can all take part in. It can be described as creative work that looks into 'stock' knowledge to devise new thought and applications to a given subject or situation. It may be primary research into a specific subject area that has not been covered before or it may reaffirm results from previous work, solving new or existing problems.

The process of 'systematic investigation' will involve looking into, probing and examining the subject/topical area chosen so it can be explored, with investigations examined and analysed, and appropriately scrutinized. So the process will involve assessment, reading and sifting through previous studies if appropriate.

So we now ask the question about research potential – what is its role and how does it play its part? Research is a process by which we gather information to look at the improvements we need to make; to answer specific questions that have arisen around the knowledge that is required to progress and improve a particular situation. Research is instrumental in problem solving but does not necessarily provide the 'final' answer – it's dynamic and can always be progressed to newer heights of understanding and knowledge that will begin to provide new development and answers to challenges that face us. Research provides:

- understanding of issues
- knowledge of the complexities we face
- workable and informed ways of working
- evaluation of success – has what's been achieved been successful in meeting the challenge?
- sound recommendations based on the empirical knowledge gained

How do we do research?

There are many systems that can be used to plan and execute a research topic, to answer specific questions and formulate the project. The following offers one approach to undertaking and planning the research, highlighting the steps to be taken:

- Identification of the research topic or problem to be addressed
- Literature search/review
- Specifying the purpose of research
- Determining the specific research question(s)
- Development of the conceptual framework – usually a set of hypotheses

- Identifying the 'method' and methodology to be used (this will inform the type of data collection)
- Data collection
- Verifying data
- Analysing and interpreting the data
- Reporting and evaluating the research
- Communication of the research findings, and, if required, listing recommendations

Research itself has been researched! Can it be made better to underpin new methodologies? Decades ago research was considered the domain of the scientists alone and its construct was based on scientific methodologies – chemistry, physics and biology as pure sciences. Research has since undergone a dynamic change into other and more varied areas of methodological approaches. Take, for example, the social sciences, which initially fell under scientific paradigms and were considered under the assumptions of science, which were based on the production of knowledge and specific assumptions – this was 'positivism'. Many assumptions, however, began to be questioned and critiqued, and it was found that it needed a shift towards methods reliant on hypotheses, which tested the positivist approach, leading it into areas of participation, collaboration and exploratory paradigms – a post-positivist area of enquiry. This leads us into the understanding of our own perspectives and thought processes. The researcher now needs to consider first and foremost their own understanding of knowledge production and the enquiry processes they base their understanding on – ontology and epistemology, words which will direct the researcher into areas and processes that they are about to engage in.

What are ontology and epistemology?

Ontology comes from the Greek 'ontos', which means being, and 'logos', meaning study. It is the study of being: the study of what exists and how things are understood and categorized – personal ontology will point towards what we think is 'real' and 'exists'. Your 'ontology' is how you answer the question: 'What is reality?' It is important, because whatever assumption you make affects how you approach your research.

While ontology deals with the sets of philosophical questions which arise when we consider the nature of reality, epistemology deals with questions about how we understand reality – about how we can make knowledge claims of any kind; how we gain our knowledge of the world, how we came to believe in a particular process or belief. Epistemology governs how we gain and adopt, for example, our 'morals'. This word comes from the Greek 'episteme', which means knowledge, and 'logos', meaning study. It is the study of knowledge and how we come to 'know'. Your 'epistemology' is your answer to the question: 'How can I know reality?'

This may now pose the question: What is the difference between epistemology and methodology? Methodology is another important consideration in research (this will be covered later); the difference, although they are very closely related, is that methodology is focused on the way in which we come to know – specific ways and methods by which we find out, in other words, the practice that is employed to find out about knowledge, whereas epistemology is based around the philosophy of how we know and come to understand what we know.

The question exists as to why this is important. As researchers we will see the world, processes and procedures in very different ways – that's what makes us who we are! However, unless we debate this in a meaningful and logical way, taking in differing intricacies and talking about them in a meaningful way, the subject becomes obtuse and will not be explored properly. Sometimes this may work and be acceptable, but without rationalizing the debate around our own 'ontology' we cannot conclude how the production of knowledge contributes appropriately to the research.

Other terminology you will come across

An understanding of these terms and processes will aid the research that is undertaken. This understanding is important when formulating a plan of research – what am I trying to achieve and how will the subject be examined to achieve the desired outcome? – an outcome that will be based on a particular question or hypothesis that needs investigation and answer. The question, though, may not be answered and may lead to other questions requiring a different approach. An understanding of the terms given below will help the researcher to decide which approach will work in a given subject or process: how the 'world' is viewed, what are the perceptions of people and processes, philosophical viewpoints (of both researcher and subjects). As time and understanding increase, this will identify how broad the subject of 'research' can be – too much to cover in one chapter, but the following will introduce the basics that need to be grasped.

Paradigm – A paradigm, in the most basic sense of the word, is a framework containing the commonly accepted views about a subject, structure or process: a structure of what direction research should take and how it should be performed. The paradigm can be described as a philosophical and theoretical framework of a principle or discipline within which theories and generalities and the experiments performed in support of them are formulated.

Realism – This is the view you will have of the 'external world' and that it exists independently of perception – the 'truth' is there whether or not you can see it or understand it. Realism is the notion of 'acceptance' that anything non-observable actually exists. A prime example is the phenomenon of a 'black hole'. Scientists have never seen a black hole, however, theory shows that they do in fact exist. There is an 'antirealist' notion that is in opposition, diametrically opposed to the realist point of view, in as much that a theory should never be regarded as the truth. It suggests that scientists and their attitudes try to ignore this debate and let philosophical deliberation decide the details of what reality is.

Positivism – An individual perception that all knowledge is based on scientific principles and is pursued by scientific methodology. In a positivist's view point, science
was the be-all and end-all of gaining fact and 'getting at' the truth. It was
science that simply 'stuck' to what could be observed and measured, and
anything else (beyond this) was unimportant and impossible to grasp.

Empiricism – All knowledge is based on what you can observe though the 'senses'. This
provides the basis of scientific methodology. That is, all evidence has a central
theme based on scientific principles that are 'empirically' based, which depends on
results that are derived through experimentation and results based on observation.

Relativism – This is the position that would suggest all points of view are equally
valid, and that all truth is relative to the individual. This means that all moral
positions, truths and culture can be understood in their own specific context and
that there are no universals.

Subjectivism – A theory of knowledge, and how it is achieved. Subjectivism holds
that knowledge is generated from the mind and personal experiences, without
reference to reality and that this forms the foundation of factual knowledge.

Social constructivism – A sociological theory of knowledge according to which
human development is socially situated and knowledge is constructed through
interaction with human beings as they interact and engage with each other.

Methods and methodology

There is a distinct difference between methods and methodology. The researcher will
need to identify exactly what they need to achieve in the enquiry and not 'jump' straight
into specific details of data collection before they have engaged with the 'larger' or
macro frameworks of specific strategies and 'grounding' of the proposed study.

Methods – The methods will dictate the techniques used to collect data and how it
will be analysed. These may include interviews, observation, etc. The analysis of
the specific data collected needs to be worked in with the type of data collection
– this leads into formulating whether it is going to be qualitative or quantitative.
These will give the researcher the **tools** or devices used to collect data: checklists, interviews, questionnaires, etc.

Methodology – This forms the framework that provides the strategies for the study,
such as ethnography, action research, mixed approach, qualitative or quantitative. Good, sound research will be seen as collecting data and analysing it within
a design that can be seen as credible, standing up to a high level of scrutiny.

Qualitative research – This involves the understanding of human behaviour and
behavioural patterns and reasons that impact on that behaviour. This means
asking broad questions about such behaviour and collecting data – words,
images, etc. – that can be analysed to inform a thematic hypothesis from a specific question. It is linked with philosophical theoretical constructs of 'social
constructionism' which is the theory of knowledge in sociology and communication
theory that examines constructed understanding of shared assumptions about

reality. It is centred on the notion that humans rationalize their natural experiences by looking at social models which are refined through language. So qualitative research is primarily exploratory, used to gain specific insights into identified problems and/or help towards the development of ideas or hypotheses by looking at trends, thoughts and opinions. Data collection methods will vary and can be structured or semi-structured, which may include questionnaires; group workshops and focus groups which will generate discussions; individual interviews and observations. Participant sample sizes for qualitative methods, as a result of the collection methodology, tend to be smaller.

Quantitative research – This involves systematic investigation of quantitative properties and their relationships by asking narrow questions and collecting data numerically. It is data and the collection of information that can be quantified and measured in number form. This data is then looked at by statistical analysis and can be used to establish a causative or associated relationship between any of the variables. This type of research is linked to a 'positivist' theoretical or philosophical stance, which is looked at through logic and interpreted through sensory experience. Verified facts and data received from the 'senses' are known as empirical evidence – this means that 'positivism' is based on 'empiricism'. Due to the nature of gathering 'exact' numerical types of information, quantitative methods do have their limitations. They do not allow for thoughts and reasoning behind the responses given by subjects or the participants in any investigation. As a result, quantitative methods are used to quantify opinions, behaviours and attitudes and can be used in larger population groups that otherwise couldn't be studied with qualitative collection methods. Collection methods may include surveys of varying designs, online polls and interviews, for example, with specific questions that are designed to collect the relevant numerical data – hence its usefulness in large populous groups.

Conceptual vs empirical research – 'Conceptual' research is that related to some abstract idea(s) or theory. It is generally used by philosophers and thinkers to develop new concepts or to reinterpret existing ones. On the other hand, 'empirical' research relies on experience or observation alone, often without due regard for system and theory. It is data-based research, coming up with conclusions which are capable of being verified by observation or experiment.

Action research – A study or studies carried out through an activity or within an occupational involvement/activity to improve the methods and approach of those involved. This type of research features frequently in education and learning institutions. It is important that action research helps educators be more effective at what they care most about. A process of enquiry undertaken by and for those who are taking part in an 'action'. It aims to assist in improving and/or refining actions taken within a specific field of work or occupation.

Mixed approach – This approach utilizes both qualitative and quantitative data. It's a term that refers to an emergent methodology that advances the systematic integration of the two within a single investigation or sustained enquiry. The premise of this type of methodology suggests that it allows a more complete utilization of data than using the separate qualitative and quantitative collection and analysis of data.

Phenomenology – This style and method of research are based around the study of 'humans' and how they experience moments and experience in life and living. This 'phenomenon' would be looked at in the present as well as interactions in the past and how these are shaping what we do now. Phenomenological research in healthcare will look at the kinds of enquiry that will address our practices as healthcare providers – the everyday, daily experiences with our patients and how we talk to and interact with them on a professional level. The phenomenological researcher would need to engage in an 'openness' to become part of and experience the phenomenon we need to understand. This, then should lead the researcher to arrive at an understanding that will contribute to our reflection on the specific topic and inform practice appropriately. This study will always be around a meaningful, experienced aspect of the subject's lived event. In healthcare this will nearly always be based around experience of how the patient was treated and cared for within a specific field of medical practice.

Ethnography – This style of research looks at and studies the social interactions of specific groups, communities or people. Teams and organizations and their cultures are examined to gain insights into the make-up, views and interpretations of that particular group. Qualitative research would use conversational interviews and discussions to probe emerging and already instituted issues. Other artefacts that would be gathered and used by ethnographers in their evidence gathering would be records of meetings (minutes), diaries and even images, for example, photographs and diagrams which would be representational of the subject matter. In healthcare, ethnographic research would be useful to gather detailed information on professional relationships in patient care and how the 'organization' responds and implements practice.

Which methodology should I use?

This is a question that can only be answered by the individual researcher and will be determined by the type of research being undertaken. The research question needs to be matched with the appropriate enquiry, which is always determined by the researcher not the methodology. Each particular research proposal and situation is unique. You will need to understand what you want to identify in the study and how the dynamics of this will affect it. With this in mind, you as the researcher will need to be fluid in your approach and adopt a particular method of enquiry to answer the question(s) being posed.

Literature

Research demands discipline, planning and a huge amount of autonomous work. It doesn't just happen by itself, but demands planning, personal commitment and, above all, persistence. A supervisor or mentor is of paramount importance in this process to aid and guide throughout the process from beginning to end. One of the most important first steps is to engage with the literature early. This is probably one of the biggest challenges at the beginning of any research project, but it will inform you of the background work in that particular area and help to narrow down your own research topic and lead to the development of the research question. Look at the literature early on as it will help to provide the independence and knowledge that will be required in your topic area as well as helping your understanding. It will also give you the knowledge required to give you an 'expert' point of view – you may become the 'expert' within this topic area.

The array of research papers and information is now more accessible than ever. There is an amazing amount which is available through the many resources such as online search engines through the internet, as well as the various library resources and databases available to search professional and academic journals, books, etc. There is no shortage of information and literature. Talk your search through with your supervisor or mentor (or librarian), who will guide your search appropriately. Good advice would be to start early and read – this will inform you and your approach to the chosen research topic and help to focus your plans and approach to answering the question.

The literature review

To gain the knowledge, and inform, it tackles to answer what you seek
It starts with the literature review

What is the literature review?

This section aims to support and help the undergraduate (or postgraduate) who may be undertaking a major project or dissertation for the first time. It may also help and inform those who, within their professional role, need to undertake a project that requires an amount of reading 'around a subject' to find specifics relating to their field of enquiry or topic being looked at to enhance better patient care.

If you are that undergraduate who is required to undertake a dissertation, then I would suggest that the first thing would be a search and evaluation of the search findings around your chosen topic or field of study. The student would be expected to show an understanding of the topic and compile a range of literature to build a 'bibliography' of relevant information, enabling them to 'mind-map' the way ahead in organizing the presented work. This would then set up the scaffolding on which this literature can inform and build, into the final written review, project or dissertation.

Objectives

There are certain objectives to think about when undertaking the review:

- **Objective 1:** Use relevant searches to seek appropriate literature in your field of study and to meet the requirements of your topic.
- **Objective 2:** There is then a requirement to start the synthesis and evaluation of the gathered information in a summary and mind map.
- **Objective 3:** Continuation of objective 2 – start to critically analyse the literature, which will help to identify areas that lack specific information or 'holes' in current knowledge and evidence-based thinking. It will show limitations in the literature and guide the formulation of further research and work.
- **Objective 4:** Present the information in a logical and organized way. The literature review usually has an organizational pattern to it, and this will help with objective 2, to synthesize and develop a conceptual theory around the topic.
- **Objective 5:** Ensure that the information and review highlight to a reader that you have an understanding of where the review fits into, and hopefully adds to, an existing knowledge base already out there, and that you have a grasp of the topic.

The student will need to demonstrate they have an awareness of the general body of knowledge that already exists around the subject under review. You need to show that learning has taken place from what has already been written and that you have made a sound analysis of the subject matter, which may lead on (hopefully) to other and new ideas.

You can now summarize the research that has been reviewed around the subject area, and make links to it through how your work has been undertaken and written up.

Important information at source

Follow these simple steps to align the work, the structure of the writing and annotation of the searches to the topic area:

- The analytical features of the literature review might provide a new interpretation of 'older' material that, once debated and interpreted, may lead to new practice.
- Follow an intellectual process that will progress the work and review the field of study to allow debate and analysis of potential 'holes' in evidence that may exist.
- This will lead to your conclusion as to identification of where the possible gaps exist and how progress has been made to identify, through the research, the specific problem and/or outcome.
- Don't reinvent the wheel – avoid researching what has already been done, or that doesn't have relevance to the area you want to develop, improve or add knowledge to, in answering your research question.

Your review will help to identify others who have written in a similar field. Gaining knowledge in this area will show you have interrogated the evidence already written about, demonstrating that you have thought about the depth of knowledge required in your review. It may also prove useful to contact various other authors to gain ideas from their perspective that will provide an invaluable source of support and help. This will put your work into perspective – are you advocating something quite new or revisiting old evidence with a view to improvement? This is essential in healthcare so new treatments or processes can be developed.

Do not fall into the 'trap' of writing descriptive accounts or lists from your reading. It is not a paper-by-paper or article-by-article list summarizing what you have read. It needs to be a piece of work that highlights to the reader what knowledge or specific ideas have been acknowledged, progressed and agreed in the area of your research that will outline the strengths and weaknesses of the project, hopefully adding to the body of knowledge to improve practice and patient care.

Structure and how to do it

You will need to ascertain and find out what is out there – read, read and read again! This is your literature search, which starts the review and project off. Once you have a topic and/or research question, you can define your search terms, ensuring you have a complete understanding of where you need to go. What are the key concepts, the key words that are required in the search? Use Boolean logic to help with the search to define the key terms and words.

Think about the search and where you are going to obtain the information. Be creative and use as many sources as you can to gain as much as possible – libraries, electronic databases, the internet, all will aid the assimilation of material from professional journals, newspapers, magazines, and of course relevant texts, to inform your bibliography. There will be other areas of information that may be relevant, such as conference papers, policy documents and reports – national and local. Remember that the most up-to-date information will come from professional journals and that textbooks, even newly published, may well contain out-of-date information.

The information gained from the various sources is very much made up from professional and specific theories based around the professional region covered within the practice area – in this case, it will be based in and around healthcare. It is usual to put everyday practices and occurrences into a specific classification or mind map that allows some logical organization or categorization. This is no different to how we need to go about categorizing our review and searches. The ideas and the way in which we need to categorize relevant searches should be progressed in the same way. Classification, at its most basic level, is all about sorting and organizing things in a logical sequence and building a mind map of where we need to be, where we are going and what needs to be done. See the suggestions for producing a mind map in Chapter 1, 'Making Sense of Essay and Academic Writing'.

Introduction

A literature review should follow the same structure as that required of an academic essay or assignment. It should begin with an introduction, defining the topic and putting the review into context, with an explanation of the scale and range of the review and a rationale for the reasoning behind it. If you are reviewing a subject or topic that is wide-ranging, you may need to explain and rationalize a specific focus. For example, if you were looking at the implementation of the World Health Organization (WHO) checklist, you may want to qualify your review by saying that your aim is to look at one particular aspect. You may say that, 'There is a large amount of work and research that has been undertaken around the implementation of the WHO checklist; however, this review is going to focus specifically on the communication factors in the "team brief" and "time out". However, as the focus is specific, the WHO checklist as a whole will only be referred to as appropriate.'

Main body/discussion

This section should be for you to discuss and organize the literature into common themes that will provide the reader with an insight into the chosen topic and the relationship between your topic and the wider subject area – e.g. the WHO checklist. You can now move the work and review, from your research, into the specific focus of your enquiry. Discuss the literature found and the critical analysis of all the literature chosen. This may take the following form, split into both knowledge and argument (from the critical analysis of the literature):

Knowledge

- Introduction and evaluation of other previous work on the topic or subject area
- Identification of what others have found and consideration of what they have seen as important
- Identification of how specifics have been highlighted by other authors and definitions developed from their work. What conclusions have been drawn from that work?

Academic argument

- From your critical appraisal, highlight what you have found to be inaccurate from previous work
- Put forward an explanation of how things may be made better and changed to increase best patient care

- A proposal for change – what may benefit the patient from change, from your research
- Disproving of a previous argument or objections that may have transgressed older arguments

Conclusion

This is an important aspect of your writing, where a summary of important information gleaned from the existing body of literature is highlighted. It forms an evaluation of current practice, policy or procedures in the existing literature. It is important here to extrapolate on the 'gaps' or 'holes' in existing knowledge that have been found, delineating where further study could be undertaken to produce better practice. Ensure that your own research is linked to existing knowledge found in your research.

Don't forget, you may need to write a chapter within your literature review on the methodology used – if this is to be used – a 'method' for a project or dissertation.

Summary

Doing the literature review is to undertake a systematic search to identify literature and past research on a given topic or specific area of practice. This literature is then appraised and evaluated to enable new insights and new areas of thought to be applied to practice, enabling better patient care and development of processes to enhance the patient's journey through their healthcare experience. It will also inform different and larger studies to answer other clinical problems that may require new ways of thinking from a critical review of previous work. The basic principles of a literature review will underpin the way in which the researcher goes about seeking relevant information, forming a basic organizational structure in line with the type of review being undertaken. The topic requires careful selection, careful searching of everything pertinent to the topic and appraisal of that information, to come to a relevant conclusion with recommendations of a way ahead for change and further research to provide a better patient journey through their healthcare experience. The literature review may be undertaken to provide better care or be undertaken as part of an academic assignment or project as an undergraduate or postgraduate scholar.

Glossary

Acculturation A term that refers to the process of adapting to other cultures – blending into the majority population (i.e. immigrants having to adopt to new customs in the country they move to). The implications, though, are that both will add to each other's cultures while maintaining their own distinct individuality.

Action research A reflective process to solve a progressive or an immediate problem, that is dynamic and will provide answers or guidelines to a particular situation. Action research looks at various forms of social actions using a cyclical approach to fact-finding and planning to gain the desired results. Fact-finding research does not necessarily have a defined, identified outcome to a particular problem, but will develop transformation towards change. It asks the question within organizations and communities of 'what can we do?' as well as 'what can we do to improve things?' in a process of change. The term 'action research' was first mentioned by Lewin in 1946 where he suggested combining theory and research that could be combined in practical problems (Gray 2018).

Artefact An academic or educational artefact that constitutes an object put together by students to fulfil a need within their learning journey. An entity that requires development and production that becomes sustained, robust and produces a visible object to display knowledge and understanding of a given task.

Authentic/authenticity To be authentic is to seek reassurance that conduct and evaluation are genuine and credible. To avoid bias by having equal access to a specific research enquiry being both valid and reliable. In qualitative research authenticity determines the rigour and trustworthiness bound by an objective and reliable foundation.

Bibliography (annotated) A list of texts, books, articles and documents to inform the reader of the relevance and quality of the sources used in a piece of work. This list of citations is usually accompanied by a brief descriptive paragraph – this forms the annotation, which will inform on the clarity and appropriateness of the inclusion.

Case study The collection, preparation and presentation of detailed information and data pertaining to a particular group or participant. Some information may also come from the subjects themselves. A study that reports on a given subject or scenario that will inform knowledge to change or improve a situation. Useful reading for evidence-based practice (EVP).

Conceptual research Research that is related to theory, thinking about abstract ideas to develop new concepts or revisit previous ideologies. It can be used to organize ideas into specific concepts and frameworks that are and become quite distinctive to apply. It can be manifested by interconnecting ideas and theories, leading the researcher to formulate these theories by using observation of self or others.

Confidentiality In research this is where no one except the researcher knows the identity of any of the participants. Information used or gained is treated with trust that it will not be disclosed to any party other than those to whom permission has been granted. It will not be revealed to others without explicit consent of the participant.

Consent/informed consent Permission gained from participants in research. This requires a research subject or participant to appreciate the current situation and nuances of what the research entails and how it may affect them. All participants must be given full and clear information about the subject being investigated and they need to understand their involvement – giving their consent to inclusion.

Constructivism This arises from the notion that reality is socially constructed. A view that reality cannot be understood outside of the way we interact as human beings and that knowledge is constructed, not discovered. Constructivists believe that learning is more active and self-directed than behaviourism or cognitive theory would assume.

Copyright A legal framework that grants the creator of a piece of work exclusive rights to its ownership, both physical and intellectual. Copyright may not be 'forever' – it may be limited by time and exclusive rights may be limited by exception.

Critical/criticality Expressive specificity of a given situation, being decisive of something that exists or information being read. It can be used when fault-finding or detracting when critically reading or evaluating an article. The adjective means urgent, important or pivotal. It may refer to crucial information in research and findings.

Culturalism A viewpoint based on a set of beliefs in a theoretical approach, showing the significance of culture in individual beliefs. Determination of how an individual or societal body reacts to and within a social and societal situation determined by their cultural background or beliefs.

Empirical Evidence or research that is based on practice or practical experience/experimentation, as opposed to theoretical supposition. Evidence that relies on experimentation rather than theory. Empirical evidence may be used to back up theory or theoretical research depending on the specific topic.

Epistemology This is concerned with how knowledge is constructed. What constitutes knowledge and how it is validated.

Ethics The moral code governing conduct, behaviour or activity based on virtues that are socially acceptable. Concepts of right and wrong conduct, providing guiding principles determining behaviour to prevent harm and do good.

Ethnography This is research concerning the study of groups and cultures. It may transpire over a given period of time where a group is observed through researcher integration within the group. This may give rise to more detailed data collection via various collection methods as the researcher is more immersed in that group or culture.

Evaluate To make a judgement about the value of an item, or the assessment of an artefact or method. To judge and inform about quality or importance of a (physical) condition in medicine. To judge merit or worth and gain insight into a specific change or initiative.

Focus/focus group This is where a small number of people form groups who are set specific tasks to examine and explore a problem or topic. They may be tasked to come up with solutions or options around that topic or question, normally guided by a leader or moderator to keep the 'focus' or flow of the investigation going forward, enabling collection, evaluation and synthesis of the results.

Grounded theory Researchers observe a group as an entity and look at how individuals work with that group. They observe how theories emerge from the observations which are grounded in the observations. The researchers add their own insight as to why those experiences occur.

Hypothesis A question or explanation based around the premise of a theory while seeking a causal action or reaction to multiple theoretical variables.

Interview Used mainly in qualitative research, a method of obtaining specific personal information to inform the enquiry. The interviewer works directly with the subject or interviewee and will probe and ask primary questions which may lead to further enquiry and follow-up questions. Obtaining first-hand information and answers on the interviewee's specific experiences.

Likert scale This is widely used in research to measure responses and opinions using various degrees of answer responses (normally 1–5 scale). It gives a more varied response than just a 'yes' or 'no' by having moderations above and below the 'agree or disagree', 'yes or no' answer. This will provide a deeper insight into thinking and opinions by providing responses such as 'strongly agree' through to 'strongly disagree'.

Meta-analysis A meta-analysis uses a statistical approach to combine and pool results from a number of different studies to answer a specific question. This is designed to increase the robustness of singular or individual studies by using statistical results of empirical research studies summarizing all the evidence.

Mixed approach/methodology Research based around the use of two or more specific methodologies from both the quantitative and qualitative research areas. It can describe the blended approach, combined approach or research triangulation.

Narrative This is a term to capture personal experience from a given period of time to inform the researcher's question. Used in interviews, it draws on experiences or 'stories' told by the interviewee which can be used to obtain objective and reality-controlled 'truth' that the researcher can analyse to create answers based on nuances such as culture, values and beliefs.

Objective(s) To state the overall aim of a particular project which will lead to an answer and a result which is sought by the researcher – what will be achieved at the end of the project or study. The objective should relate to the question, hypothesis or identified problem.

Ontology The study of being. It is the study of what exists and how things are understood and categorized – personal ontology will point towards what we think is 'real' and 'exists'. Your 'ontology' is how you answer the question: 'What is reality?'

Paradigm A system of belief or theory that informs what we do. It tells us of the knowledge being developed and how this relates to the views and question initially identified. The paradigm will guide the researcher through a decision-making process and how the research is carried out. It establishes the practices, ranging from thought to actions.

Phenomenology Qualitative research undertaken to examine a 'phenomenon' or how human behaviours are perceived and understood. The researcher can look into the perceptions and understanding of those who have experienced a specific situation.

Plagiarism A practice of passing off someone else's work as your own. Not acknowledging others' work when citing or using it in your own work.

Positivism This is set within a scientific philosophy which argues that only scientific research can deal with observable phenomena directly from clear and precise observation. Observation and experimentation are used to influence and directly explain theory.

Qualitative methodology This is exploratory research, obtaining an understanding of reasons, opinions and motivations by looking at trends and thoughts to observe particular problems or questions – this may then feed into the formulation of further ideas or hypotheses. Common methods of data collection would be interviews, focus groups, questionnaires and specific observation.

Quantitative methodology This research methodology is used as a technique where the problem being looked at is quantified by the collection of numerical data that can then be transformed into usable statistics. This is a much more structured approach which uses measurable results and data to examine particular patterns in research. Quantitative research uses multiple forms of data collection which can be directly measured: surveys, online polls, detailed questionnaires and systematic observations. The Likert scale is an example of a data collection tool.

Random sample This is a basic sampling technique to choose a select group or population of research subjects. Each member of the sample group is selected randomly, completely by chance and anonymously. Each selected member has an equal chance of selection, which provides a completely unbiased select group of research participants.

Range The difference between the highest and lowest in a set of data.

Reliable/reliability The quality of the research data and information must be able to be trusted. Making the research measurement tool reliable must be prioritized prior to use. Reliability is important to minimize the variables, keep the research valid and ensure the results of the study are robust and stand up to scrutiny.

Research A systematic investigation into a study, to answer a theory, hypothesis or specific investigation, to determine facts and develop new learning and knowledge.

Research tool These are the methods used to gather data and information during your research project. Another name is a research instrument – these may be interview schedules, questionnaires, video recordings or checklists. They are instruments to help with task accomplishment.

Sample/sampling The type of analysis and the research tool being used will determine what type of sample will be required, e.g. a predetermined questionnaire with a set number of observations or a Likert scale with specific questions. See also 'random sample' above.

Subjectivism This is a theory that suggests there in no truth outside of the individual's own experience. It also purports that truth is subjective and is very much dependent on the individual's own mind, thoughts and experience.

Systematic investigation This is the concept of study and investigation using a methodical approach, for example, setting the question or hypothesis, defining the methodology, valid and reliable data collection and conclusion.

Systematic review This summarizes the results of sound and well-designed studies or controlled trials. Used in healthcare, it provides a high level of effective information and research findings into many healthcare interventions, which allow and inform patient care recommendations. As an example, evidence-based practice uses these reviews to inform new practice and treatments/patient care.

Triangulation A useful technique which is a powerful validation tool in research, used to check and cross-check data from two or more different sources. It will test the consistency of research findings and remove causes of invalidity which may influence the results. This may involve multiple researchers acting independently or using different research tools or theoretical schemes to quantify the data.

Validity If the research measures what it is supposed to, it is said to be valid. This is a term to determine how well a 'test' measures what was intended. The test can be reliable but not valid – conversely it may be valid but not reliable. In summary, validity means that a test or investigation is accurately measuring that which it's supposed to.

References and further reading

Bowling, A. (2014) *Research Methods in Health,* 4th edn. Maidenhead: Open University Press, McGraw-Hill Education.
Gray, D. (2018) *Doing Research in the Real World,* 4th edn. London: Sage.
Green, J. and Thorogood, N. (2014) *Qualitative Methods for Health Research,* 3rd edn. London: Sage.

4   Evidence-Based Practice: Why Do I Need to Understand, Read and Apply It?

This chapter is designed to aid the understanding of and emphasize the importance of evidence-based practice (EBP) for practitioners as a basis for and in clinical practice. The student or practitioner will be able to apply the appropriate means for the identification and retrieval of evidence relevant to their own clinical practice. It will describe EBP and the range of methods used for research in healthcare, and its importance to the use of research and relevant evidence to aid patient care.

A common and succinct definition of EBP comes from Dr David Sackett:

> the conscientious, explicit and judicious use of current best evidence in making decisions about the care of the individual patient. It means integrating individual clinical expertise with the best available external clinical evidence from systematic research. (Sackett 1996)

Increasingly, clinicians and medical staff from all professions are being challenged in their delivery of healthcare and treatments. The general public has become and continues to grow more knowledgeable about the specifics of medical problems and their respective treatments. This knowledge comes from numerous sources – televised media, social media and the internet, to name but a few. As a result, if they fall ill, patients question and 'test' the medical professionals, requiring whatever medical intervention is deemed necessary. So as practitioners we need to achieve a strong and supportive, patient-centred approach to their care using the most up-to-date and current evidence available to allow us to give answers and support without breaking the patient's confidence in our practice. Considerations will need to be based around key principles of healthcare ethics – beneficence, non-maleficence, autonomy and justice.

These principles need to form the basis of all our practice. Healthcare education aims to teach, support and provide a high quality of care that is based on the best and most current evidence available. It is therefore incumbent on the student to understand this in their studies, and more importantly to understand the need for its continuation once qualified.

The student developing skills and learning evidence-based practice will need to gain the confidence to initiate conversations, reading and choosing the relevant research and information, identifying and retrieving evidence and outlining the importance of such evidence-based practice in their own clinical area.

There are numerous definitions assigned to 'evidence-based practice' in the literature. One that seems to sum it up well is offered by Barker (2010), who, following Sackett (1996), defines it as:

> the conscientious, explicit and judicious use of theory-derived, research-based information to make decisions about care delivery to individuals or groups of patients, taking into consideration individual needs and preferences.

What needs to be in the minds of all healthcare practitioners is that evidence-based practice integrates problem-solving, systematic and critical thinking approaches to determine an answer to any important clinical question which may affect the healthcare of any patient or patient group.

Evidence will come from many sources, and as such needs to be grounded in substantiated seminal texts that are of high quality and peer-reviewed as sound research. It is therefore essential that students (and qualified practitioners) have the skills to evaluate relevant evidence, its strength and appropriateness. It therefore becomes essential to have a greater understanding of research, and what is good empirical research and what is only 'media-centred' unsubstantiated research. In the United Kingdom, the body that informs on evidence-based practice and recommendations in healthcare treatments is the National Institute for Health and Care Excellence (NICE). This body sets standards and guidelines in medical practice based on proven research that has been scrutinized appropriately.

There are more than 3,000 medical journals on one medical search engine alone, with more than 6,000 to 7,000 articles or papers being added weekly. All studies are not equally well designed or interpreted, which requires critical analysis to understand which of those are sound, as against those of a lesser value or rigour.

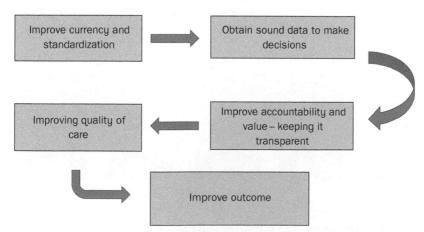

Figure 4.1   Evaluating values – improving practice

This explosion of evidence needs careful assessment and evaluation to gain the best information to facilitate best patient care.

It is therefore important to understand the basic concept that needs to be addressed to obtain value within healthcare systems. Evidence-based healthcare must add value and improve practice (Figure 4.1).

Undertaking evidence-based practice

The student (or practitioner) should by now understand the need for and value of EBP. Consideration of your skills will now provide the opportunity to undertake assessment of relevant data and information or to assess individual areas requiring further knowledge or skills. A logical system could be used to evaluate what is required and how to undertake the necessary appraisal. First, there will be a need to define what evidence is required, based on practice and why it is important.

ASK a question based on clinical need, building a clear and answerable question, which may come from the patient or an issue arising from the care of the patient.

ACQUIRE: now search for the best evidence to help with the question and need. This is where it is important to understand the differences in research models – the difference between qualitative and quantitative research, for example, and why systematic reviews are important and why they should be a cornerstone of quality evidence.

APPRAISE the evidence and judge whether or not it is reliable, and critically appraise the evidence determining its value as substantive.

APPLY the evidence and act on this in practice.

ASSESS: this is important as it's where the evaluation and assessment of the performance take place to determine its effectiveness in change and patient care.

These are described as the five steps of evidence-based practice (Figure 4.2). A spirit of enquiry should now be developing in the practitioner's mind. Without this

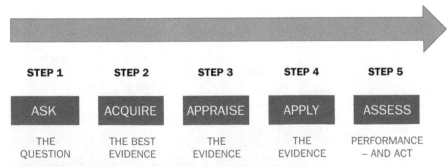

Figure 4.2   The five steps to evidence-based practice

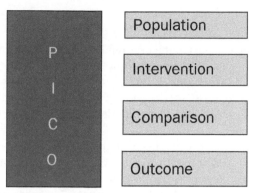

Figure 4.3 Pico diagram

spirit and willingness to see the best for our patients, the EBP process is likely to falter and not happen. Misconceptions about EBP that it's not required or too difficult to achieve need to be expunged, otherwise the 'I've always done it that way and it doesn't need to change' will always flourish and continue to do so.

To help with focusing on the clinical question, which needs to be directly relevant to a particular patient or patient problem, the question must be phrased in a way that helps facilitate an answer. The mnemonic **PICO** helps to focus on this process. It will also help to expedite the search strategy, aiding specific concepts and identifying issues that require research to answer the question (Figure 4.3).

Patient, population or problem? – How would you describe a group of patients similar to yours – what are the demographics, pre-existing conditions? What are the most important characteristics of the patient? What is the condition, procedure or disease process requiring research?

Intervention – What main intervention are you considering? What do you want to do with this patient or population/group?

Comparison – What are the main alternatives being considered, if any – different treatment approach, drug, procedure, surgery, etc.?

Outcome – What are you trying to accomplish, measure, improve or affect? What are going to be the relevant outcomes that may affect quality of life – side effects, complications and changes in clinical status, for example?

PICO can be further added to, changing the mnemonic to PICOTT with the addition of:

Type of question – Therapy / diagnosis / harm / prognosis / prevention – looking at these specifics if applicable.

Type of study – Systematic review / randomized control trial (RCT) / cohort study / case control, etc.

Study design

The type of question can lead to the best type of study design to answer it – some common examples could be: diagnosis, how to select and interpret certain tests, which may well lead to prospective, blind comparisons or cross-sectional studies. Randomized control trials (RCTs) or cohort studies would provide answers to such questions as: how to select treatments that do more good than harm and are cost-effective?

This knowledge is important when trying to answer questions and looking for specific information or research to answer them. Know the study design and this will allow you to find answers to the question.

It is important to understand study designs to enable good and reliable retrieval of the best information to answer the question:

Descriptive studies/case series and case reports – consist of collections of reports on the treatment of individual patients or a report on a single patient. Because they are reports of cases and use no control groups to compare outcomes, they have little statistical validity.

Cross-sectional studies – describe the relationship between diseases and other factors at one point in time in a defined population. Cross-sectional studies lack any information on timing of exposure and outcome relationships and include only prevalent cases.

Case-control studies – studies in which patients who already have a specific condition (cases) are compared with people who do not have the condition (controls). The researcher looks back to identify factors or exposures that might be associated with the illness. They often rely on medical records and patient recall for data that might be associated with the illness. These types of studies are often less reliable than randomized controlled trials and cohort studies, because showing a statistical relationship does not mean that one factor necessarily caused the other.

Cohort studies – identify a group of patients who are already taking a particular treatment or have an exposure, follow them forward over time, and then compare their outcomes with a similar group that has not been affected by the treatment or exposure being studied. Cohort studies are observational and not as reliable as randomized controlled trials, since the two groups may differ in ways other than in the variable under study.

Randomized controlled clinical trials – carefully planned experiments that introduce a treatment or exposure to study its effect on real patients. They include methodologies that reduce the potential for bias (randomization and blinding) and that allow for comparison between intervention groups and control (no intervention) groups. A randomized controlled trial is a planned experiment and can provide sound evidence of cause and effect.

Systematic reviews – focus on a clinical topic and answer a specific question. An extensive literature search is conducted to identify studies with sound methodology. The studies are reviewed, assessed for quality, and the results summarized according to the predetermined criteria of the review question.

A meta-analysis – will thoroughly examine a number of valid studies on a topic and mathematically combine the results, using accepted statistical methodology to report the results as if it were one large study.

Qualitative research – answers a wide variety of questions related to human responses to actual or potential health problems. The purpose of qualitative research is to describe, explore and explain the health-related phenomena being studied.

EBP – an important and integral part of the toolkit of the practitioner in healthcare. The topic will enhance both scholarly learning in undergraduate, postgraduate and continuing professional development, as well as direct action in clinical practice – providing an understanding about what evidence-based healthcare is and is not.

References

Barker, J. (2010) *Evidence-Based Practice for Nurses*. London: Sage Publications.
Sackett, D.L. (1996) Evidence based medicine: what it is and what it isn't, *BMJ*, 312(7023): 71–2.

5   Critical Thinking

The mind reacts to what it sees – look closely and see reality and the future!

Introduction

This is a term or process that will present itself in many, multivariate forms and fits within all aspects of the roles in healthcare. Understanding of our nature and how we react to learning and experience all need consideration – or thought! Getting the thought process right is fundamental to everything we do. We need to ensure that all our encounters, whether they are social, domestic or work, are 'thought' through clearly, to provide precision and clarity. Never accept what is read or seen at face value – critical thinking is about the evaluation of what we see, read or experience and questioning that information.

This can be conceptualized through Bloom's Taxonomy, which shows there is more to thinking and learning than just memory-retentive systems of learning. The top three levels of analysis, synthesis and evaluation arguably give us the higher-level thinking skills required; this is further developed by the next lower levels of comprehension and application, which allow us to understand facts and ideas and apply that acquired knowledge.

Question the ideas and look closely at the various arguments to rationalize them – especially in your studies. As a student there is a fundamental need to be able to think critically about every aspect of your studies and practice – thought processes about the information received, and how it relates to the learning and development required, are fundamental to progression into a qualified practitioner (and beyond!) As a healthcare student, you must understand the need, and your right, to ask questions and rationalize the work of others; this will inform your own writing by showing the ability to consider various arguments and viewpoints to inform your own opinions and theories. This is critical thinking – the ability to question and interrogate learning with an open mind.

Six steps to critical thinking

Critical thinking involves skills that require the use of analytical and creative dispositions in the individual – that is someone who can, by their nature, think or act in a particular way. They are inherently curious about the world, interested in relevance and able to understand the limits of knowledge, looking for probable causes and points of view as opposed to definitive proof.

Generally, people base their thinking and generation of knowledge on previous situations or experience, which is built into a cognitive thinking base to provide a baseline knowledge. The revised edition of Bloom's Taxonomy (Anderson and Krathwohl 2001) suggests a change to the levels or steps – they are now: Remember, Understand, Apply, Analyse, Evaluate and Create.

This, though, may not provide a 'best solution' to a given problem or situation requiring decision or action; previous experiences may influence thought because other parameters such as emotion may affect the decision process. The 'emotion' or affective domain of thinking would bring in the way individuals react emotionally – how emotions and attitudes affect feelings and personal awareness. This is particularly relevant in healthcare, as it impacts on how we see and react to patients and their treatment.

Critical thinking, therefore, should prevent us leaping directly to conclusions, as it should guide our thinking through particular and logical steps to gain a wider perspective and to help with the consideration of all the given 'facts'. Critical thinking can be aided by the application of different steps. Look at the provided **knowledge**, what the problem is, and has there been an attempt to solve this? What is inherent in this problem that needs to have a solution and why does it need to be solved? Now there needs to be a move to **comprehend** and understand a given situation. The problem should by now have been clearly defined and identified, and relevant information, evidence and data collected. The next step continues from the last into **application**, which builds on the evidence found, clearly addressing it to the problem that requires answering from your understanding of the situation. Looking at all the evidence and how it is linked now takes us into the **analysis**. Here we start to link evidence and data to the main problem, which should lead to identifying the situation more clearly. It involves breaking down information into its component parts to gain clarity, relating it to, or connecting it to, other ideas. Once the problem has been analysed and the evidence has been fully considered, the next step of **synthesis** starts to piece together everything that been considered and analysed, to come up with an answer, original idea and clear way ahead. At this final stage, all the thinking, analysis and consideration of evidence, data and resources that has been interrogated so far should result in an action plan, built from a full **evaluation** of the problem or instance that was initially generated. Always evaluate at the end of this critical thinking process – this avoids rushed judgements and emotional 'creep' taking the place of reasoned arguments (Figure 5.1).

A tool that could prove useful in this process is the 'SWOT' analysis, which is used to evaluate both internal factors and experiences as well as external factors.

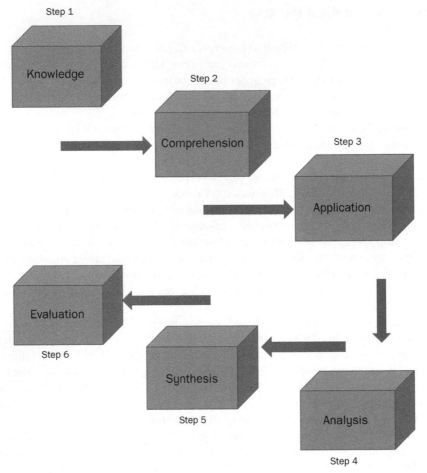

Figure 5.1 Six steps to critical thinking

Internal factors would be drawn out from the strengths and weaknesses, while the external factors would be taken from the opportunities and threats (Figure 5.2).

- **Strengths:** Thoughts and characteristics of a project, theme or event that give it an advantage over other situations or instances.
- **Weaknesses:** Thoughts and characteristics of a project, theme or event that place it at a disadvantage relative to other situations or instances.
- **Opportunities:** Areas of identification that the project or situation could utilize to its advantage and improve the situation.
- **Threats:** Areas of concern within a project or situation that could give rise to alarm, cause trouble or anxieties.

The SWOT analysis can be a useful model but it has its own weaknesses. It could lend itself to the user compiling lists rather than allowing a rational thought pattern

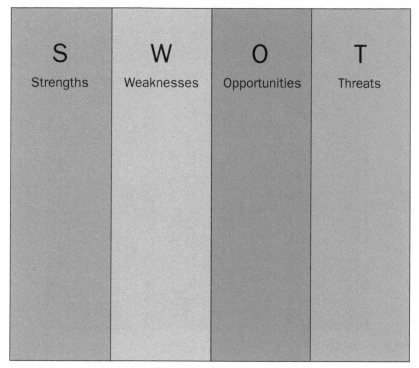

Figure 5.2 SWOT analysis

to emerge from its use. Using SWOT in conjunction with other models may avoid this and will help to provide objective rational or critical thinking. Lists alone will show an element of *'uncritical'* thinking without clear rational thought. A good SWOT analysis will produce valuable strategic information that can be used with a strong structure of thinking, whereas a SWOT that produces lists will be seen as unimportant and weak, unable to enhance the thinking around a particular project or investigation/study.

Uncritical thinking can be aligned to 'tabloid' understanding – a belief in what is read at face value without hesitating to ascertain validity, accuracy or truth – taking for granted that 'it's written in black and white' so it must be true!

It's important to understand how the uncritical thinker perceives themselves and what they do – we have all been guilty of this at some stage in our lives: they get annoyed at what is said or problems that occur, resulting in being impatient. They make assumptions based on first impressions of a given situation, focusing on their own opinions. Without *thinking*, they pretend to know more than they do, looking at ideas and solutions based on their own opinions only. They are emotionally guided rather than adopt a rational understanding of the situation with an unbiased approach.

This type of thinking must be avoided as best you can – especially in a health-care profession where the results of what we do, say and act on will affect patients in our care. So let's start thinking properly (Figure 5.3)!

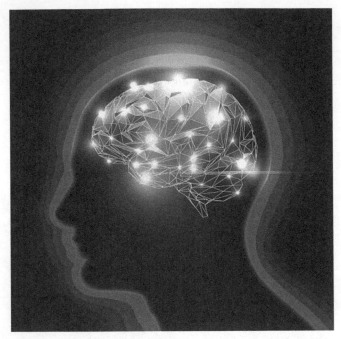

Figure 5.3 Get your brain thinking!

For the healthcare student

The healthcare individual or team should be able to use critical thinking skills not only in analysing situations, projects or journal articles for their studies, but also as they come into daily contact with patients. Teams need to utilize these skills, for instance, in the perioperative environment when undertaking the daily World Health Organization (WHO) operating theatre brief prior to the day's operating list, and the case-by-case checklist prior to the start of each surgical procedure. All healthcare professionals, which include ODPs and other professionals allied to medicine, work collaboratively with each other to ensure the patient is given optimal care. This care is based on critical thinking in its many guises and situations of use, and therefore it is an essential tool in the practice of all healthcare professionals, not just in educational or other studies. It is therefore incumbent on institutions educating healthcare students to include elements of learning and teaching on critical thinking to enhance the disposition of students and their critical thinking skills – how to explore views and evaluate alternative, unbiased evidence to enhance patient care. Students need to be taught this early in their learning career so they will be able to develop effective skills in practice; this can then be carried into their career as a qualified practitioner. Healthcare systems are developing these skills with the providers of care. This will aid the optimization of patient care, providing a usefulness not only in the healthcare provider's toolkit, but also allowing them to develop how patients think critically about their own care.

By adopting a 'critical' approach to thinking about all aspects of life, not just singularly around our particular profession or work-related subjects, we also need to consider with scepticism the 'modern-day' spam that is seen all too often. This relates to the quality of both written and verbal/observational evidence requiring consideration. How often have we seen and heard about 'fake news'? The written word that has been falsified to sensationalize and attract media attention with no real substance or truth, some of which at first sight looks both genuine and compelling. The critical thinker will, and should, see through this and if any doubt exists, will undertake some research to either validate or disprove it. Emotional judgements will produce a reactionary response to looking at the given evidence – judgements could and will be formed instantly on the available evidence presented at a given time. Take a breath, sit back and consider the evidence carefully, trying to be objective about what is presented. This objectivity is fundamental in any walk of life, but is essential when we research evidence and new thinking in healthcare. Students must start to adopt this methodology early in their learning career so it becomes second nature in both their academic work and professional practice, which ultimately will carry through to qualified practitioner status.

Questions that the critical thinker may ask to aid in the recognition of sound evidence, providing a logical model to prevent reactionary, emotional and biased thoughts, might include:

1. **How** is the evidence presented and does it make logical sense?
2. **What** has been presented and does it fit within a recognizable model or framework – is it relatable to other work or situations?
3. **Why** should I take this as a true and quality piece of work or evidence – can it be substantiated?
4. **When** is an answer or action required as a result and do I know enough about this topic to make a rational decision?

There may not be answers to all these questions, and indeed other more relevant questions may become apparent as a result of the evaluation of the evidence. What is important is the thought process undertaken which should be calm, unbiased and of a sensible length of time to make decisions about its validity and reliability. If there is still doubt or uncertainty, then you must go in search of further evidence, reading and research to help with that decision or action plan.

Putting this information and these skills into context will give you a fighting chance of understanding and engaging with a subject or topic and making a sound, confident judgement, through evaluation of the evidence, leading to quality reasons for specific opinions and actions. This will have been achieved through enquiry, analysis, comparison and reasoning and **not** through reactionary, emotional or biased lack of understanding.

Scepticism in healthcare

Do we trust all knowledge, or do we question?

This subject is wide-ranging and makes interesting reading when linked to critical thinking. There has been a great deal written on the subject and differing thoughts have been put forward which will engage the student who has an interest in this area, both philosophically and culturally. In healthcare, scepticism becomes important when introducing innovation and new practices – the need for questioning is evident and some may be sceptical and require substantial evidence to reassure them that it's the correct thing to do.

Scepticism is a widely used term that means we question what we know, what we are told, and what we are taught. Is there a place for scepticism in healthcare? There are a number of arguments and practices that we question, or need to question, in healthcare practice, to attain the best possible outcome. The theory of scepticism can be said to be that we know nothing about the world in which we live and practise; that it is motivated by an insistent individual motivation that suggests that the very possibility of knowledge and what we think and know about the 'real' world are brought into question. This scepticism is also necessary in healthcare education so that the knowledge taught and developed is in fact the best, most up-to-date and correct. The sceptics would question this, using the philosophical approach to ask about the certainty of this knowledge. In healthcare, this would be classed as local scepticism, which is specific to the questioning of healthcare-related knowledge. This can be augmented by a methodological scepticism that would question and scrutinize information and knowledge by looking at the 'true' and 'false' claims to allow transference to best practice. Therefore, the sceptic could claim that there is no absolute belief that could be achieved; there is always a demand for the validation of truth and knowledge. This is particularly important in healthcare as all treatments, interventions and new practices will be questioned and require validation to afford best practice. It could be argued that there is a role for scepticism within all new practice, as this development requires careful thought, audit of knowledge and potential outcomes in every phase of the development debate, including sceptical questioning. This, however, still requires that any scepticism would need justification – the sceptic cannot just challenge with a 'throw-away comment' such as 'how do you know?' or 'why?' Like all evidence towards any change, it must be justified and supported by rational argument and evidence.

The early philosopher Descartes and his ideas were considered to be revolutionary and radical. He was one of the first philosophers to question the existence of the world through sceptical doubt. He tried to manifestly understand knowledge through scepticism, although he revisited his beliefs as he progressed through his meditations. Scepticism was given high importance as it was used as a method to reach a level of certainty in life. He maintained his scepticism to introduce the 'I think, therefore I am' argument. He continued his knowledge investigation to find certainty and disregard all doubtful ideas. The result of the first meditation he published was the uncertainty of the senses, memory and the body. He stressed that the only thing that is certain is scepticism. Scepticism is about belief and individual perception, which Descartes highlighted (in much more depth than is reported here), but it set the scene for how this branch of philosophy would impact on our lives and knowledge. This is important when we consider our pathway through healthcare and the development of practice – what we do now and in the future. It enshrines within us the need to keep an open mind when looking at new developments and practice that will ultimately affect our patients.

References and further reading

Anderson, L. W. and Krathwohl, D. R. (eds) (2001) *A Taxonomy for Learning, Teaching, and Assessing: A Revision of Bloom's Taxonomy of Educational Objectives*. Boston, MA: Allyn and Bacon.
Bloom, B.S., Engelhart, M.D., Furst, E.J., Hill, W.H. and Krathwohl, D.R. (1956) *Taxonomy of Educational Objectives: The Classification of Educational Goals*. Handbook I: *Cognitive Domain*. New York: David McKay Company.
Cottrell, S. (2017) *Critical Thinking Skills*, 3rd edn. Basingstoke: Palgrave Macmillan.
Descartes, R. (1641) *Meditations on First Philosophy*. Reprinted in *The Philosophical Writings of Descartes* (3 volumes), trans. J. Cottingham, R. Stoothoff and D. Murdoch. Cambridge: Cambridge University Press.

6 Learning about Learning: Modifying and Maximizing a Process – Why Is It Important to Know How to Learn?

What we know is not the end – adapting knowledge gives us the edge!

What is learning?

This is about being adaptable; knowledge already held is not always the most up to date and usable. It is about having the ability to utilize, maximize and apply an enquiring mind to existing knowledge with an ability to learn and progress this knowledge. This sits comfortably with what we have talked about already in relation to evidence-based practice.

Much of the healthcare professional's life, both as a student and as a qualified practitioner, will revolve around the ability to learn continuously to achieve a specific aim – primarily around patient care. There are many tools that can be used to achieve this continuous learning – textbooks, research articles/papers from relevant journals, experience and tuition from 'experts' in the field, all of which can be substantive or anecdotal. All are equally important resources, but must be put into context.

What needs to be achieved by the 'teachers' is to maximize learning, resulting in retention of knowledge to allow a meaningful delivery of care. Teaching needs to be a discussion, interesting and compelling enough for the student to learn and to aid retention. This teaching will come from many sources – university lecturers, tutors, work colleagues and peers, and not just from those who can be considered 'formal teachers'. The delivery of this learning needs to be as described: meaningful, a discussion, interesting and compelling to aid retention and application in practice. Learning therefore will take place when we grasp a mental or physical understanding of a subject that allows interpretation of knowledge, understanding of the subject and interpreting a newly acquired comprehension of a specific topic.

Thinking is not just the main fundamental aspect of learning; learning involves many attributes that form a matrix that will contribute, involving personal senses, emotions, beliefs, understanding and values. This then helps to meet a personal need and willingness – if we don't have the will to learn, we will not be able to learn, and anything that is taught will not be secured in our consciousness.

The OASIS learning cycle

There have been many models and attempts produced to explain and show the learning process. And both academics and others have attempted to explain the learning to learn process. As with reflective practice, a cyclical approach may be used which is based on a repetitive series of instructional, thought and practical processes which help to procure an understanding and ease of interpretation; this will therefore aid understanding and consequently support learning. The OASIS learning cycle is one model that would be relevant for all types and styles of learning.

The OASIS learning cycle is made up of five steps:

- **Obtain** – Gaining new knowledge from a theoretical aspect, and/or skills or new proficiency from a practical aspect.
- **Apply** – Putting into practice the newly acquired knowledge or skill and applying the new learning.
- **Study** – Looking at and evaluating the results of practice and applied new knowledge, assessing as appropriate.
- **Interpretation** – From the assessment and evaluation, reflecting, clarifying and transforming the application and practice of new learning.
- **Synthesis** – Interrogating, evaluating and modifying accordingly, to combine all that has been learned from the original new knowledge and shape it further to enhance if required.

Similar to reflective practice, the OASIS cycle then continues and repeats to further enhance learning and application (Figure 6.1).

Theories of learning

Much research has been undertaken over the years to study the ways that individuals learn. There have been many varied theoretical proposals to describe the theories of learning and their processes. These myriad theories have broadly fallen into five main categories:

- Behaviourist
- Cognitivist
- Constructivist
- Experiential
- Social, contextual

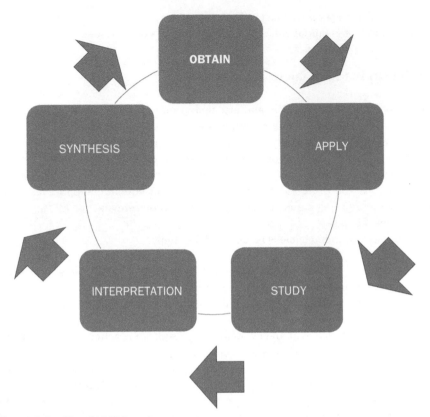

Figure 6.1 The OASIS learning process

Behaviourist

In behaviourist theory, learning is seen as a change in behaviour due to some external experience. The learning is brought about by a person being subject to some external stimulus, environmental change or experience, which causes a change in the person's behaviour. This demonstrates learning.

Behaviourism is particularly important and significant in healthcare education, where simulation is used as a learning tool. Simulation allows learning in practical skills in a safe environment without undue pressure on the student or learner, as no harm can occur (as with a real patient). Objectives that require learning will be described and identified as a specific practice or behaviour, and will normally be shown through a 'show, tell, demonstrate and do' situation. This method shows what needs to be learned, what needs to be achieved (through demonstration), and through student participation gives them the opportunity to undertake and practise the task once shown. Learning through this theory will be seen as desirable as it normally has a reward attached – this is generally through robust feedback to the learner. An example of this style is the way that computer games offer reward (praise) for good progression through the various levels of the game, or punishment by the lack of progression – this is behaviourism.

Therefore, the main feature of behaviourism is that learning will be observable, making it easy to collect and quantify information and data. Key features are thus based on observable behaviours. Criticisms of the theory include the inability to describe in detail the learning achieved, and the lack of cognitive-specific input.

Cognitivist

The paradigm of cognitive psychology purports that learning is an internal process which depends on the learners' capacity to learn, their motivation and personal determination. This learning comes from the individual's mental capacity and activity that memory, thinking, motivation to learn and reflection ability depend on.

A cognitivist learner will focus on what is taught – information given by an 'expert' in the subject to the learner who does not know. The learner will need the ability to take in the information (receive it), comprehend what has been taught and later retrieve the information from memories to enable relevant actions. The mind of the learner is likened to a filing cabinet, where the relevant drawer is opened to retrieve information that is required for action, when needed. All knowledge and information 'stored' through memory are being continuously connected, giving meaningful outputs from what has been taught. Cognitive learning can therefore be broadly looked at as a process that will be influenced by internal and external processes to instil individual learning. If this process is adopted by a learner who has a leaning towards working in this way, then the acquisition and 'storage' of information and knowledge work well. There can be a problem, however, when this process of cognitive learning becomes fruitless or difficult, as there will be learning delays and this will give rise to problems in retention of information and knowledge.

Constructivist

The constructivist will generally construct their own understanding and knowledge of experiences. The learner experiences and reflects on those experiences to gain an understanding and retention of this knowledge. Constructivist teaching will inspire learners to assess how an activity is helping them gain an understanding of an issue – this is a constant process that will revisit a topic to help the learner construct their understanding.

Any new taught information will be resolved and merged with previous ideas and experiences that may change what is believed – either enhancing the new knowledge or dismissing it as irrelevant or immaterial. The constructivist will create their own knowledge by asking questions and assess the known through exploration. Constructivist learners will visit and revisit their curiosity about what will work and how things work. This is not a reinvention of knowledge, but an attempt to gain understanding of how things work and function by applying existing knowledge. Constructivist learners, therefore, become involved by applying their existing knowledge of real experiences – they learn to surmise and hypothesize by testing theory and manipulating conclusions from the findings to better both themselves and others.

Experiential

One of the main proponents of experiential learning is David Kolb. Kolb developed his experiential model, recognizing that people learned through experience rather than just through a pure cognitive model. The experiential model consists of a four-stage cycle, and any stage of the learning process, can be accessed followed by looping through the cyclical stages (Figure 6.2). This is different from constructivism and behaviourism as it's designed to allow the learner to take a more holistic view of their experiences and to cognitively draw information and conclusions to apply in the testing stage of the cycle.

In this theory, Kolb argues that learning involves the acquisition of conceptual ideas that can be applied in a flexible way to a wide range of situations. This makes this model a useful tool in healthcare learning, as many situations are different and continuously changing. This is due to the impetus for development being provided by new and differing experiences.

- **Experience** (concrete): an experience (new or existing) is encountered
- **Reflection** (observation): it is important to understand the experience, observe and reflect – are there any inconsistencies that relate to the understanding of the experience?
- **Conceptualize** (concluding, learning from the experience): reflection giving new ideas – what has been learned from the experience – is there a modification of an existing concept that can be applied?
- **Experimentation** (testing and applying the learner's ideas): what is the new outcome going to provide, what is going to happen?

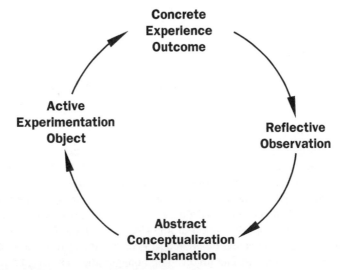

Figure 6.2   Kolb's experiential model

Effective experiential learning will be observed when a learner progresses through this cycle of learning, which can be 'dipped into' at any stage of the cycle and followed through.

In summary, then, experiential learning involves (1) having a concrete or definitive experience, which is followed by (2) observation and reflection on the experience, leading to (3) formation of concepts or analysis of the conclusions, which will then lead to (4) testing of the concepts and an understanding of the outcome(s) and testing the new experience for the future. The cycle then starts again.

This type of learning is of particular use in healthcare education and learning; it is current and uses different concepts of experience to fit a particular situation with patient care, as all can be different:

- Assessment and accreditation of learning from care and work experiences
- A sound way of facilitating change in structure and treatment in healthcare
- A sound basis for clinical supervision, group and team working to raise or change an aspect of care
- A method to increase individual awareness and development – becoming more effective

Social, contextual

This is learning within a group or community setting as opposed to individual learning. It is a shared process, taking place while observing, working together as part of a larger group that may include other colleagues or students from various backgrounds and with varying levels of experience.

Social development theory has formed much of the foundation of learning through cognitive development – the work of Vygotsky (1987, cited in McLeod 2018) has become known as the social development theory, which stresses the role of social interaction in the development of learning.

In the adult concept, the *More Knowledgeable Other* (MKO) refers to someone who has a better understanding or more ability than the learner in particular processes, tasks or concepts. In adult education the assumption is that the MKO is a tutor, teacher or older, more experienced adult – however, this may not always be the case. In many instances, the 'younger' person may be the individual who has more knowledge or experience. This can be seen in the younger person's knowledge of computing or computer gaming, for example. Who owns more knowledge in these areas, the older adult or the younger student? Some learning methods employ electronic support systems and don't rely on a person at all – an example being the mandatory training undertaken by healthcare staff, which is ostensibly an online learning resource. The key, therefore, to the MKO (or electronic teaching program) is that they must have more knowledge than the learner about a particular topic.

Vygotsky coined the term 'scaffolding' to describe the various forms of support that educational providers can offer learners; this came from his social development theory. This 'support' might include verbal teaching, questioning, suggestions and directions, all aimed at increasing the breadth of a learner's activity where the learner cannot accomplish this alone.

Social learning also follows in the 'role-playing' scenario, which is an example of a social and contextual forum – role plays are multilayered and involve team working, again important in healthcare education, especially simulation. This learning is important as it represents instances of social support, encouragement and a 'scaffolding' for learners to improve their performance, knowledge and experience without the worry of doing something wrong with a live patient.

It will be clear by now that individuals will learn though various models and processes, some of which won't be understood and they will just happen to fit the situation at hand. Models that can be followed can be used to structure, plan and deliver/receive successful learning opportunities. Learning is something we all do, all of the time from early childhood to ageing adults – 'we are never too old to learn' – even though it may not be realized, it is something that is happening.

Applying learning principles in healthcare education will probably involve changes to help transform perceptions of individual roles within this field. Adopting a differing view of both learner and facilitator to meet each patient's care needs may well be required, and the key institute or educational delivery unit may well need to embark on cultural, educational and operational changes to meet the requirements. The clinical environment is a challenging place for learners, and also for the educator, as interaction and facilitation are required to meet needs and changes to perceptions, views and beliefs – as the care and treatment of a person are at the end of this process. Because of this, it is important to maximize learning input to facilitate the best use of learning theories when aiding this learning process.

The clinical teaching and learning environment is an ideal area to utilize adult learning theories. This helps to reinforce logical and clear thinking, and their consideration should be fundamental to improving clinical learning and outcomes.

References and further reading

Jarvis, P., Holford, J. and Griffin, C. (2003) *The Theory and Practice of Learning*. London: Routledge.

Kolb, D.A. (1984) *Experiential Learning: Experience as the Source of Learning and Development*. Englewood Cliffs, NJ: Prentice Hall.

McLeod, S.A. (2018) *Lev Vygotsky*. Retrieved from: https://www.simplypsychology.org/vygotsky.html (Accessed November 2019).

Vygotsky, L.S. (1962) *Thought and Language*. New York: Wiley.

Vygotsky, L.S. (1987) Thinking and speech, in R.W. Rieber and A.S. Carton (eds) *The Collected Works of L.S. Vygotsky, Volume 1: Problems of General Psychology*. New York: Plenum Press (Original work published 1934), (pp. 39–285).

7   Presentations: Saying What You Mean and Meaning What You Say

A successful presentation is just a conversation

Preparation

In many aspects of our learning the delivery of a presentation of one kind or another will be expected. From student life, having to produce a presentation, either individually or as a group, through to the need, once qualified, to be able to present information to others in a team or to management reporting on a study, audit or practice. Presentations take many different guises; they may be PowerPoint presentations or just a brief verbal report back on a topic or relevant subject. For example, in the operating theatre it may be that you lead the team briefing to your individual theatre staff, or in a ward environment, to the nursing team at change of shift, to name but two instances. Therefore, the sharing of your studies, work and achievements is an essential part of the role we all have in healthcare as both students and practitioners. The experiences as a student will form sound practice for when qualification and ultimately more senior posts/positions are sought and achieved.

Engaging with the audience is paramount – trying to convey enthusiasm and a mature demeanour will serve you well and help to detract from minor errors and nerves. You will want to keep the audience engaged – interaction helps to get the audience closer to understanding and embracing your ideas. This helps to show them that you value their input, engagement and connection with you the presenter.

Rationale

Presenting information clearly and effectively is a key skill in getting your message or opinion across, and today presentation skills are required in almost every field.

A presentation is a means of communication that can be adapted to various speaking situations, such as talking to a group, addressing a meeting or briefing a team – or, with relevance to our professional area of practice, talking to the theatre team.

To be effective, step-by-step preparation and the method and means of presenting the information should be carefully considered to fit with the need, type of presentation required and the reason behind its relevance.

The presentation

There are many tools available to the presenter, and they should be chosen to meet the needs of the presentation to be delivered and the particular audience. These range from flip charts, white boards, slide projectors, etc. (Figure 7.1).

The most commonly used tool for presentations is PowerPoint. There is an art to using this program; it should not be used to compensate for a lack of clarity in your presentation and the information you are trying to deliver, but the slides should complement your delivery, defining clearly the message that you are trying to convey. This should be worked out prior to the completion and writing of the slides.

Keep the design and development of the slides simple; presenters have a tendency, at times, to overcomplicate them by cramming in too much information in a small font. Try to avoid slides that are too fancy – graphics and illustrations are good, but they must be succinct and relevant. If using bullet points, no more than four, maximum five, should be used on each slide.

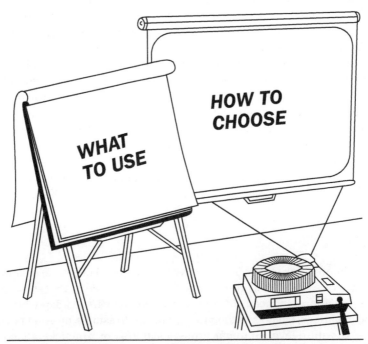

Figure 7.1   Choosing the tools for your presentation

Keep the number of slides small, as it's important that the audience listen to you and not spend their time reading the slides – too much information on multiple slides will cause the audience to lose concentration.

Do not read and look at your slides – the slides you project to the audience are not your notes. If you read directly off your slides, then you may as well just give them a written sheet. Remember, the audience wants to listen to you and not see the back of your head while you read off each slide.

Ensure your slides can be easily read – dark text on a light background is best. Try to avoid a white background as this may show too much contrast, and avoid fancy fonts that may prove difficult to read. If you have prior knowledge of anyone in the audience who may be dyslexic, then choose a coloured background and font suitable for them – this may involve prior conversations to find out what is going to be best.

Use key words and try to avoid using full sentences on the slides, as these take time to read and may interfere with your own verbal presentation.

Ensure that when you prepare the presentation, the information and subject(s) flow. Often when you are preparing a presentation, the information is all there but it's not in the correct order as you were in a hurry to get down your thoughts. Go back into the slides and go through them, ensuring they flow and are all in the correct order of delivery.

Deliver your presentation to the audience – remember you are talking to people from all backgrounds and knowledge levels; you are not just talking to the back of the room. Maintain good eye contact with everyone, use your hands appropriately and remember that it's good to walk around, within reason, within the confines of the room. Do try to avoid 'rattling keys or loose change in the pockets' and other nervous twitches that may annoy.

Do not be frightened to use anecdotes of relevant stories to help with audience engagement – it adds to the interest and keeps them focused on you. Invite audience participation through questions and answers all the way through the presentation as this, too, keeps audience participation high and maintains the interest you want.

Practise your presentation

Begin in an empty room and pretend you are giving your talk to an audience. If you have time, present it to a friend or colleague(s), and ask for feedback. Time yourself – timing is obviously important if this is a consideration – student presentations will have a time limit.

Identify potential obstacles

Practise answering tricky questions you think you might be asked; try to anticipate these and have a plan in the back of your mind to cope. Rehearse words you find difficult to pronounce. Also try to plan for IT problems and issues – have back-up data sticks and alternative presentation artefacts in case of electrical IT failure.

On the day

Take everything you need with you (for example, pens, slides, props). Arrive before the audience and test the equipment. Go to the washroom. Check that you look the part. Wash your hands or splash water on your face if you feel sweaty or flushed. Then return to the room and welcome the audience into your space.

Keep the audience interested

- Use a flip chart to write down the audience's contributions to aid feedback.
- Show or draw pictures or diagrams.
- Show a video.
- Give the audience tasks individually, in pairs, or in groups.
- Bring a patient with you, if appropriate.
- Use props or models.

Coping with presentation nerves

It is entirely natural to feel nervous before making a presentation! Many seasoned teachers, lecturers and other presenters feel nervous beforehand, despite having given hundreds of presentations. The same is true of others working in the media or in the public eye. Being nervous is **not** a problem or a weakness; you just need to channel your nervous energy wisely. On the other hand, being overconfident and not nervous could be a weakness!

When you feel nervous before a presentation, the following strategies and exercises should help you.

Practise deep breathing

Adrenalin causes your breathing to become shallow. By deliberately breathing deeply your brain will get the oxygen it needs and the slower pace will trick your body into believing you are calmer. This also helps with voice quivers, which can occur when your breathing is shallow and irregular.

Drink water

Adrenalin can cause a dry mouth, which in turn leads to getting tongue-tied. Have a glass or bottle of water handy and take sips occasionally, especially when you wish to pause or emphasize a point. Take care not to take large gulps of water.

Chew gum

Chewing gum before a presentation may help you to feel more relaxed. Research has shown that the act of chewing can increase your alertness and help to reduce anxiety. It is best to get rid of the gum before you start your presentation.

Smile

Smiling is a natural relaxant that sends positive chemical messages through your body. Smiling and maintaining eye contact also help you build rapport with your audience.

Use visualization techniques

Imagine that you are delivering your presentation to an audience that is interested, enthused, smiling and reacting positively. Cement this positive image in your mind and recall it just before you are ready to start.

Self-massage

Press and massage your forehead to energize the front of the brain and speech centre.

Pause

Just before you start talking, pause, make eye contact, and smile. This last moment of peace is very relaxing and gives you time to adjust to being the centre of attention.

Slow down

Speak more slowly than you would in a conversation, and leave longer pauses between sentences. This slower pace will calm you down, and it will make you easier to hear, especially at the back of a large room.

Move around

Move around a little during your presentation, as this will expend some of your nervous energy. However, try not to pace backwards and forwards or rock on your heels, as these activities can be distracting to your audience.

> **Stop thinking about yourself**

Remember that the audience is there to learn some information, and that it is your job to give that information to them. Try to put your nerves aside and think about communicating your message as effectively as possible.

You are 'on', even when you are not speaking

In a team presentation, *everyone* is being watched, not just the presenter. Therefore, stay alert, listen and show an interest in what is being said. Remember, your body language can convey a positive or negative message. Stifle that yawn. Don't slouch or look bored, and unless it is absolutely necessary, do not whisper an aside to another team member. Also pay attention to the audience; you may pick up signs that will help you to gauge audience response. That can be useful if you have yet to present! Remember, to be successful as a team presentation, it must come off as just that: a *team* presentation.

After the presentation

Give the audience relevant references, invite questions, and if you're unable to answer any questions, then take details and say you will get back to them with the answer.

People who ask difficult questions often do so to show off their knowledge. These 'questions' often begin, 'Isn't it true that …', or 'But what about …', and can often be 'answered' by simply thanking the questioner, as these are not really questions to you the presenter. Alternatively, ask the questioner for their opinion. They will probably be happy to expound on the subject, as this is the reason they spoke up originally.

Get some constructive feedback from the facilitator or a trusted colleague.

Now you can congratulate yourself – it's over and you succeeded. It is easy to focus on what went wrong, but you should now look at the positive aspects, making sure that you engage these for the future in other presentations you may have to give. Forget for now any aspects that did not go well, but try to remember them for the next presentation you give.

You may not find that following this advice decreases your anxiety or nervousness, but the experience will only serve you well for the future as it should get easier, and you will start to enjoy making presentations. You will achieve a certain 'feel good factor' from doing this.

8   Student Engagement and Engaging with Fellow Students: Peer Support Using Individual Experiences in a Student Group

'Been there, done that – I can help you if you haven't'

Student peer engagement

Within a cohort of students, there is always a mixture of experiences and knowledge owned by different students. Peer support is when these students share and provide this knowledge to their student colleagues. Students engaging with fellow students will continue to provide a very useful support mechanism within a cohort as they can provide knowledge, social and emotional support, and practical help to each other. The 'peer' is a person (student) who is fundamentally the same as the next person. The relationship between them is seen as one of equality in the social sense, but one may have knowledge that the other does not have – he or she may have 'been there, and done that' and can pass this on and relate to others in a similar situation on a notional similar level.

Engaging with each other in this way will enhance team working and working together, sharing experiences for the greater good. In healthcare, this is important, as collaborative working is fundamental to good practice. Engagement in this way is about focusing on how to get students to care, both for each other and for the recipient of their knowledge and care – the patient. It will give them motivation to understand concepts independently and to share this understanding and experience as a result.

Creating a study group

One of the strategies for the encouragement of peer-to-peer learning is the formation of study groups. There is normally group work associated with any course, which will, as described already, encourage team working and collaboration – preparing for their roles as qualified healthcare providers. This can encourage students to be more invested in the course content by being interactive within it, therefore helping to facilitate better grades and outcomes. It also provides the ability to organize and develop skills in leadership and management – important skills that will be required in any healthcare career and future work.

The reality of any study group is that there will be those who are keen to collaborate and engage and those who will come along 'for the ride' and be happy to be led and allow others to do the work. Most university students are placed into groups by the course tutors and have to try to collaborate as best fits the given group. If the opportunity exists to select group members, which is not beyond possibility, then some pointers can help develop the dynamics of the group and ultimate collaborative working:

Choice of contributors: Look for the students who will aid the success of the study group. By now the class will have worked together for some time and an awareness of characters and their learning and social culture will be evident. Note those who exhibit a desire to learn, who listen and take notes, participate in discussions in the class sessions and contribute actively. Do not discount the quiet and shy students, though, who still exhibit a desire to learn but remain quiet in class. They can add to the group as this shy persona may be helped in a smaller, more private group; they may also have a wealth of knowledge and experience that is not overtly obvious, but will come out in a smaller group.

Shared aspirations: These aspirations will obviously be around the topic or subject the group has been given to develop. Discuss what each group member has to offer and what can be gained from each individual in the group; each student will have various experiences that could prove imperative to the group dynamics. Ensure the ultimate goal and end point of the group do align to allow collaborative working, so all members can work together to meet the goals.

Group rules: Setting some ground rules is important to ensure the group focuses on the task. The group needs some basic guidelines to avoid it becoming a social event and discussions going astray from the main point and purpose of the group and its ultimate achievement. It would be prudent to set a timetable of expectations, meetings and venues; agree a delegated task for each member and what they will bring to the group and what they will do within a set time scale. With this in mind, it would be useful to have a form that is completed at every group meeting that highlights what needs to be done, by whom and when completion is achieved.

Figure 8.1 shows an example of a group record that could be adopted and modified for recording group meetings and work.

Peer engagement to maximize learning – online

Online learning can be utilized in many ways, and can offer advantages to those for whom classroom attendance is either difficult or impossible. Most learners now are computer- and IT-literate and will be able to adapt to this way of learning very easily. Help and support from fellow cohort members allow engagement with the whole class if an individual cannot attend for whatever reason. This type of engagement can

Group Meeting Record		
Record of group meeting discussions (notes). Task:		
Meeting date	Hand in date	
Meeting chairperson's name	Chairperson's signature	
Names of group members	Signatures of group members in attendance	
List of topics discussed		
Task agreed	By whom	By when
1.		
2.		
3.		
4.		
5.		
6.		
Date of next meeting		

Figure 8.1 Group engagement record

also be used for study group work, as remote engagement can be facilitated through interactive programs such as Skype or WebEx. Skype-to-Skype calls are free anywhere in the world and can be used on a computer, mobile device or tablet. WebEx provides an online meeting and video conferencing facility.

This type of collaboration allows students to have connection with their peers to assist them with class-related issues where accessibility of a particular text or research paper is 'out of reach'. Connecting through email and online discussion groups can be a method of sharing information and articles. The online discussion groups can be through social media groups set up for the particular cohort in question and every member can be given access. This needs to be policed carefully as it could descend to just a social 'chat' – just like the study groups, guidelines need to be agreed.

Using this technology is useful in most cases, but it depends very much on knowing as much as possible about the students, their capabilities in this field, and how confident they are and what experience they have in the 'digital' world. This can be gained by profiling the students at the beginning of their course or enrolment.

Student engagement – why this matters

It is well recognized that students learn better when they are actively involved in their learning. Students themselves are also more likely to be engaged if they feel and know that they are being actively involved in the design and shape of what they are being taught. It also means that working in partnership with students to create and evaluate learning designs, including digital designs, helps collaboration.

For tutors and lecturers who only have limited experience of technology, working in collaboration enables them to enter the 'students' world'. Collaboration can also remove misconceptions about the choice of learning, helping students to understand what they will learn and gain from independent and collaborative learning – both online and face-to-face. Lecturers and tutors are able to learn from the students to provide the best approach and methods for student engagement and learning. So engagement is not just peer-to-peer but tutor-to-student and student-to-tutor as well.

Modifying or changing the nature of how students learn and engage within the classroom may provide a variable and workable solution to aid them with their achievements and goals. However, changing the nature of the classroom and its learning structure may not help some students who are perhaps lacking in certain skills and understanding of the specific learning strategies required. This is where collaborative engagement with both tutors and peers is important, as various strategies can be adopted to aid understanding and ultimate mastery of these goals and skills from both directions.

A culture that empowers student engagement

The importance in any institution, now, to encourage and empower student engagement, is to create a recognizable and transparent culture that gives the students a 'voice'. The educational institution members and their students should take a lead together in establishing this culture, providing a process that can be helpful in providing benefits to both parties. Students will have a different perspective on what is expected, what they need to be taught and how this will give them the skills and knowledge to be able to undertake employment with the relevant qualification. Some members of the teaching staff may have reservations about this type of collaboration, but this needs to be discussed overtly and honestly with sound demonstration of roles.

Student engagement may also lead to a greater mutual respect as it will give students a greater awareness of the teaching staff's workload and expertise – that they are not just there to deliver a teaching session occasionally, but they do have a myriad of jobs/roles to undertake in between. On the other hand, the teaching staff need to understand that the students are advocates and fee-paying customers looking to maximize their educational experiences and outcomes, to fulfil a career aspiration. Student voice is powerful and important, as it should be.

> Listening to and understanding what students express will profit all and produce a valued insight into their world and psyche.

This mutual cultural collaboration is important, as both students and tutors will realize that when their opinions and values are heard, it will enhance understanding and the reasoning as to why certain decisions are made. It may go some way to showing greater tolerance for unfavourable experiences and decisions that do not seem beneficial; the outcome is that constructive feedback, debriefing and debate can and should take place.

9   Ethical Principles in Healthcare

To show respect to others is a mirror of your moral self

What is ethics?

To students and practitioners the term 'ethics' will be a consideration in all aspects of care and education, and will form an important part of the development and learning in these areas, both as a student and qualified registrant. Ethics is a moral philosophy that is involved in the ordering, preserving and endorsing of the concepts of right and wrong. It is often required that disputes of a moral nature are addressed to seek both clarity and resolution. Ethics, therefore, plays an important part in the life and career of any healthcare practitioner, both as a student and after qualification, as it is an area of study that looks at moral behaviour and how people should act. There are individual nuances that are required as a student and a healthcare practitioner, but the principles are the same. Every person is expected to represent themselves with honesty and respect, whether this is by the written or verbal word. These principles rely on the representation of honesty and respect to provide only truthful material information at all times. Therefore, ethics is the rules we use to establish what is right and wrong in our lives. Normative ethics is the determination of a 'norm' of ethical rule that underpins ethical behaviour, while applied ethics is the application of normative ethical beliefs to real-life issues in everything we do.

Ethics in education

Academic honesty expects that all students maintain the highest standards of integrity in every aspect of their student time. Work that is not the student's own work, that has been created by another and not acknowledged, will receive no reward or credit. This is an act of lying and deceit and is tantamount to theft, and will be seen as such. This is plagiarism and is the taking of someone else's work and passing it off as your own; those who plagiarize are committing serious legal and ethical violations. Ethical values in education are essential as they set the standard of acceptability: what is acceptable and what is not. This protects the interests of both the educators and the students. Educational ethics is applicable to both the educators and students – it is the educator's role to make the students aware of the principles, and it is the institution's management responsibility to ensure educators are familiar with these principles and that these are relevant to their respective profession.

Teachers, tutors and lecturers play an important role in a student's development. They not only deliver knowledge but also develop the personality and professionalism of the student, especially if the course of study is leading towards a registerable award. In this respect, the educator will play an important role in the mentorship of that student. They will aim to influence either overtly or covertly the student's development towards this professional outcome that is essential for their practice. Educational ethics that is applicable to educators requires them to show patience to all students irrespective of their learning abilities. Every student should be treated equally and given due justice while taking an action. It's important that an educator understands that every student is different and shouldn't be evaluated on the same basis. Ethics in education does not allow educators to hold grudges and to treat students unfairly. At the same time, ethics in education requires a student to respect their tutor and to abide by the rules set by them. Students should acquire academic integrity and responsibility as well as practise self-discipline. Ethics in education helps regulate the education system and ensures that this practice positively contributes towards human welfare – this is important in healthcare with patients.

Morality

Ethics provides us with a method of understanding morality. In its basic form, morality refers to the differences between right and wrong. Morality itself will give us many standards which we will inherently have learned about, throughout life development and growing up. Everyone who leads a 'moral' life will abide by accepted rules that are readily understood. We will know the difference between right and wrong; we know that to kill, lie and steal, for example, are wrong, and remain happy in this philosophy and are accepting of this. Both education and healthcare hold inherent moral standards, some of which have already been discussed and would be seen as the norm. Professional morality, like normal morality, has a set of standards, but professions also have moral norms for their practices. This is apparent in the healthcare profession. For example, the rules surrounding consent and medical confidentiality are specific to that profession and are not generally appropriate outside of medicine.

Principles of healthcare ethics

While the role of healthcare practitioner can be rewarding, it can also be challenging. For any practitioner delivering patient care, the procedures and treatments have both downsides and advantages. Patients have a say in their treatment considering certain circumstances and personal inputs. Guidelines developed by

Beauchamp and Childress (2013) help to make decisions when a difficult and complicated situation arises with patients. The four principles of healthcare ethics are *autonomy, beneficence, nonmaleficence* and *justice.*

Autonomy: In medicine, autonomy refers to the right of the patient to retain control over their body. A healthcare professional can suggest or advise, but any actions that attempt to persuade or coerce the patient into making a choice are violations of this principle. In the end, the patient must be allowed to make their own decisions – whether or not the medical provider believes these choices are in that patient's best interests – independently and according to their personal values and beliefs. This can sometimes be difficult when the patient is a child or person with a learning difficulty.

Beneficence: This means to do good. This principle states that healthcare providers must do all they can to benefit the patient in each situation. All procedures and treatments recommended must be with the intention to do the most good for the patient. To ensure beneficence, healthcare practitioners must develop and maintain a high level of skill and knowledge, make sure that they are trained in the most current and best medical practices, and must consider their patients' individual circumstances; what is good for one patient will not necessary benefit another. However, the practitioner must not forget that the patient also has autonomy and has the right to refuse treatment or interventions.

Nonmaleficence: Simply means do no harm. This principle means do not do anything deliberately to harm or injure a patient or make them worse than they are. However, sometimes harm will occur, such as a reaction to drugs or medical treatment – iatrogenic harm.

Justice: The principle of justice states that there should be an element of fairness in all medical decisions, an equitable use of healthcare resources, fairness in decisions that burden and benefit, as well as equal distribution of scarce resources and new treatments, and that medical practitioners should uphold applicable laws and legislation when making choices.

Case study example (hypothetical)

A female patient has a kidney growth that, if left untreated, will result in kidney failure and ultimately a diagnosis of cancer. An operation to remove the growth/kidney is the best treatment, especially to make a firm diagnosis, but the patient is frightened of needles and is against having surgery that would require a needle to give her an anaesthetic. The medical team and anaesthetist must work with the patient to respect the fact that she dislikes needles and doesn't want the operation (her **autonomy**), and they need to find a solution that would prevent her from going into kidney failure and possibly later stage cancer, which is in her best interest (**beneficence**). Although the surgery is the best choice, forcing the patient to accept the needle would be harmful to her (**nonmaleficence**). Finally, the medical team and anaesthetist need to consider the impact that the patient's choices might have on others if she starts to go into preventable kidney failure – or worse, she will need dialysis, which affects other people who need the same treatment (**justice**). Therefore, before making the final decision the doctor must consider all four principles of healthcare ethics, which will help the medical team make the choice that will have the greatest possible benefit for both the patient and society.

References and further reading

Beauchamp, T. and Childress, J. (2013) *Principles of Biomedical Ethics*, 7th edn. New York: Oxford University Press.

Berglund, C. (2012) *Ethics for Health Care*, 4th edn. Melbourne: Oxford University Press.

Strain, J., Barnett, R. and Jarvis, P. (eds) (2009) *Universities, Ethics and Professions: Debate and Scrutiny*. London: Routledge.

Index